HERBAL REMEDIES

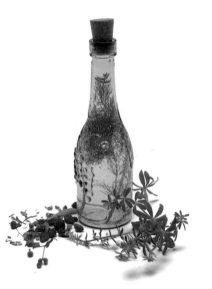

TAMARA KIRCHER and PENNY LOWERY

PETER ALBRIGHT, M.D., SERIES EDITOR

MACMILLAN • USA

A QUARTO BOOK

MACMILLAN
A Simon and Schuster Macmillan Company
1633 Broadway
New York, NY 10019-6785

Library of Congress Cataloging-in-Publication Data

Herbal remedies / Peter Albright, consulting editor.
    p.   cm (A Naturally better book)
   ISBN 0-02-860834-8
   1. Herbs Therapeutic use Popular works. I. Albright, Peter,
1926– II. Series: Naturally better books.
RM666.H33H472 1996
615′.321—dc20   95-37892
                           CIP

The book was designed and produced by
Quarto Inc.
The Old Brewery
6 Blundell Street
London N7 9BH

Senior Editor Sally MacEachern
Editor Alison Leach
Indexer Dorothy Frame
Senior art editor Penny Cobb
Designer Alyson Kyles
Picture researcher Susannah Jayes
Illustrators Elisabeth Dowle, Wayne Ford, Sharon Smith
Photographer Paul Forrester
Picture research manager Giulia Hetherington
Editorial director Mark Dartford
Art director Moira Clinch

Typeset by Central Southern Typesetters, Eastbourne
Manufactured in Hong Kong by Regent Publishing Services Ltd
Printed in China by Leefung-Asco Printers Ltd

10 9 8 7 6 5 4 3 2 1

CONTENTS

This book is not intended as a substitute for the advice of a health care professional. The reader should regularly consult a health care practitioner in matters relating to health, particularly with respect to any symptoms that may require diagnosis or medical attention.

INTRODUCTION

Flowering plants first grew on this planet about 135 million years ago, rapidly evolving into the main groups of plants we recognize today as a result of their differing environments. Farmers who work with traditional methods say that animals know instinctively which plants will be good for them when they are sick; whether this was also the case for the predecessors of the human race, or whether they used trial and error to ascertain which plants did them good and which were harmful or even fatal, there is no way of knowing. Inevitably, though, humans have always had a close relationship with plants, using them as they evolved for food, clothing, rope, shelter, and medicine, and to feed their animals.

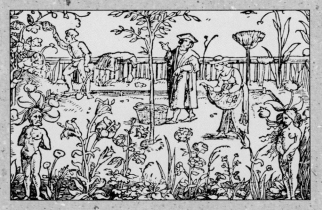

Traditionally, the herb garden with its roots, leaves, flowers, and berries provided inspiration for health and wellbeing.

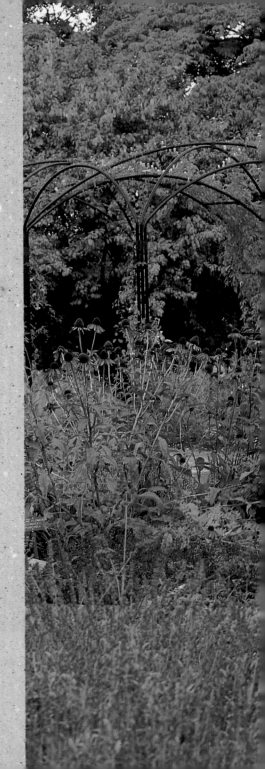

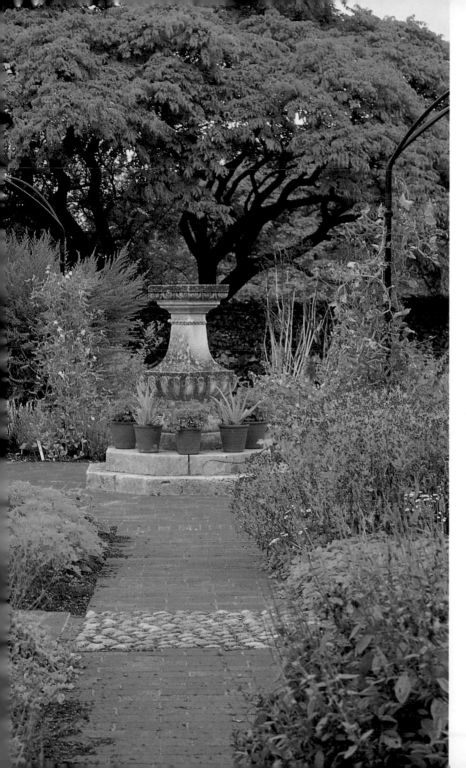

It is thought that the earliest written record of the medicinal use of plants dates back to the Sumerians who described the use and actions of thyme, among other remedies, over 5,000 years ago. The earliest known Chinese herbal, compiled in 2700 B.C., lists 365 medicinal substances and their actions; many of these are still in use today, notably Ma Huang (*Ephedra sinica*), from which the modern drug ephedrine is derived. Even Psalms in the Old Testament has some herbal knowledge to impart: "Purge me with Hyssop, and I shall be clean." The Egyptians of 1000 B.C. are said to have used cilantro, mint, garlic, and other plants for food, dyes, and medicines; and some fundamental principles of healing were expressed by the Greek and Roman medical writers. Hippocrates recommended fresh air, rest, and improved diet combined with herbal remedies to restore health, whereas Galen saw the remedies he proposed as a complete system: he included not just plants, but medicines derived from animal and mineral sources, as does the classical system of homeopathy. These early Greek writers describe herbal medicines supporting the person's "life force." This concept is similar to the ancient Chinese concept of *Qi* or *Ch'i*, terms which usually mean "energy," but can also mean "air" or "breath." *Qi* is an essential element of Chinese medicinal theory defining the difference between life and inertia or death. The Greek idea of life force also corresponds to *Ki* in Japan, which means the vital force flowing through the body.

The more formal herb garden offers peace and tranquility through the beauty of its scents, colors, and design.

At times in the past, magical properties have been attributed to herbs and those who knew about them; this naturally gave rise to superstition, fear, and suspicion, and ultimately the persecution and death of many wise women, healers, and witches. Of course, some ancient uses of herbs sound like nonsense to us today, and perhaps some of them were completely ineffective: Avicenna, an Italian philosopher of the Middle Ages, recommended a method of contraception in which the woman would drink large quantities of infused basil – *not* to be tried! It was generally believed, in the same historical period,

Many important herbs, such as echinacea and false unicorn root, were part of the extensive herbal tradition of the Native Americans.

that the root of the mandrake plant shrieked when it was pulled out of the earth, causing insanity followed by death to anyone who heard it. The plant was considered valuable as an anesthetic and expectorant, however; so the bizarre practice evolved of tying a dog to the stem to unearth it!

Not all medieval herbal practices by any means were ineffectual; early surgeons used a sponge soaked in opium, henbane, hemlock, mandrake, and ivy which was held close to the patient's nose to inhale, thus deadening the pain of amputation or surgery very effectively. Of course, these herbs are all highly toxic, which meant that if the unfortunate patient breathed the cocktail in too vigorously, he or she was likely to overdose and expire.

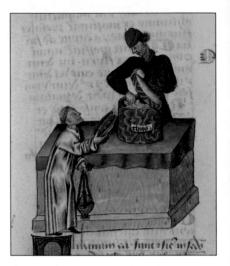

Garden thyme, derived from the Greek word "thymus," meaning courage, was used in medieval times to invigorate and to inspire strength and bravery.

HERBS AND THE ENVIRONMENT

Even though little written herbal lore has been inherited from the Native Americans, their use of herbs for healing and rituals is well known through oral records. The discovery of many important herbs like echinacea is thanks to them. Native Americans emphasize the need for people to live in harmony with their surroundings. It has long been the tradition of many tribes, when they take something from the Earth, to compensate by giving something back to her. If all cultures had this principle, our planet might not be threatened by deforestation, intensive farming, and over-industrialization. Perhaps because of their all-important relationship with "Grandmother Earth," Native Americans have given us knowledge of, and access to, some particularly valuable herbs for the reproductive

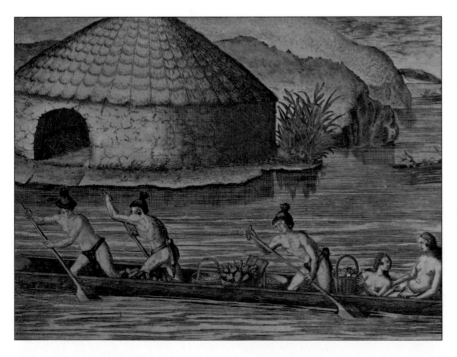

system; for example, false unicorn root, which is mentioned in the section on reproduction and urinary problems (see page 40).

Users of herbs are fortunate today: not only do they inherit the wisdom of many cultures to provide them with knowledge about the historical use of plants, but also laboratory investigations have been able to isolate the multitude of chemicals which occur naturally in herbs, enabling people to know what they are good for and why. Some of these constituents are necessary to the life of the plant; a great many, however, are not, which suggests that these natural medicinal substances have been provided for human beings by the planet, to help to sustain life and health. There has probably been more continuity in the use of herbs as medicine than in any other method.

The choice of herbs that is now available, with the help of modern infrastructure, is quite extraordinary. Herbs that grow in China and Japan, Europe, Africa, and the Americas can be obtained in other areas; whereas our forebears were limited to those that grew in their own neighborhood. Ironically, intensive farming methods have reduced the availability of herbs that grow wild in the countryside – frequently, they are seen as weeds and destroyed in favor of crops. Furthermore, many people live in cities without access to gardens. This need not be an obstacle, however, with commercial sources of herbs, and even mail order, becoming more accessible to everyone.

Until very recently, the manufactured drugs prescribed by doctors were all derived from plants: aspirin from willow and meadowsweet (whose botanical name, *Spirea*, it has borrowed), steroids from wild yam, ephedrine from *Ma Huang*. Some drugs are still synthesized from herbs. This fact may be what saves some parts of our environment; pharmaceutical companies have been known to buy areas of land to prevent its destruction by loggers, as has happened in part of the Brazilian rain forest, in order to make sure that specific plants with medicinal ingredients will still be available. The result of extracting one or two active constituents from a plant, however, is to produce a drug with an isolated action, thus losing the balanced energy of the herb, which originally had many actions that worked holistically on the human organism. Another result of producing chemical drugs in a laboratory is the associated pollution of the environment by toxic waste products; using herbs medicinally has no such negative implications – it means working *with* the environment, not against it.

HERBS AND LIFESTYLE

Herbs are very effective as a way of caring for both our bodies and our psyches, but they will work best if you look after yourself on other levels, too: if you eat well, exercise gently but regularly, try to breathe fresh air (when available!), and find ways of dealing with stress, the herbs will have a more harmonious environment with which to work. Although herbs can help with some emotional problems, anyone who is very anxious or distressed, or has unresolved issues from the past, is advised to seek counseling or psychotherapy.

Many herbs are also eaten, either as flavoring or as an intrinsic part of a dish: garlic, fennel, ginger, parsley, thyme, sage, and basil are good

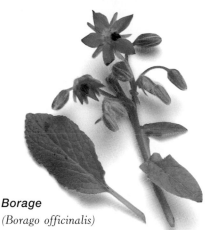

Borage
(Borago officinalis)

examples. Some herbals also list foods such as lemon, onions, and leeks, and specify their medicinal actions; and extract of lettuce is included in some nervine relaxants for its sedative properties.

It is possible to see food and herbs as part of a continuum, with food that has no medicinal action at one end, moving through the area where herbs and nourishment combine (including culinary herbs and medicinal food), to plants which are only used medicinally. At the extreme end of this continuum, there are the herbs which are actually toxic when taken in large amounts, but in smaller quantities may be healing for tumors and other serious conditions, which are of course beyond the scope of this book.

It has been said that being a good herbalist is very similar to being a good cook; prescriptions are just another kind of recipe! Of course, not all herbal mixtures taste good, but everyone knows that good food can benefit our health.

KEY HERBS

There are probably more than 2,000 medicinal plants available worldwide – an overwhelming number for the novice herbal user to grapple with! So here is a manageable quantity of herbs which are commonly used, easily available, and safe for most occasions. There is no need to buy all of them at once; you will build up a stock gradually, as you need the different herbs. Remember, both tinctures and dried herbs keep best when stored in a cool, dry, dark place. In many cases, fresh herbs can be used, if they are available; you will need to use slightly more by weight, to allow for their higher moisture content.

As we mention in the section on *Basic Principles*, it is usual to mix several herbs together, which gives a broader range of actions than using just one herb. As far as we know, all herbs are compatible with each other and mixing them together can only enhance their healing properties. The table of recommended dosages on page 19 will apply whether you are taking one herb or several, and tinctures mixed together will keep just as long as single tinctures, provided you protect them from sunlight.

In this section, we have given a brief description of the medicinal actions of each herb, the part which is used, and some examples of ailments it is used to treat. We suggest that, when you have found a herb or combination of herbs in the *Specific Applications* section, you cross-check their description here to make sure they are suitable.

Echinacea
(*Echinacea angustifolia*)
Also known as purple coneflower, Kansas snakeroot, comb flower, black Susan, hedgehog, and Sampson root, its botanical name comes from the Greek *echinos*, meaning hedgehog, which its flowers resemble. The Native Americans have employed this extremely useful herb for generations to help clear microbial infections, both bacterial and viral, and boost the immune system. It is widely used and combines well with many other herbs, being effective for respiratory tract infections, cystitis, catarrhal conditions, acne, and infected cuts or wounds. It has a reputation as a natural antibiotic, with none of the unfortunate side effects of antibiotic drugs; historically, it has also been used to treat rattlesnake bite.
PART USED: root

Nettle
(*Urtica dioica*)
This is the common stinging nettle, which grows wild all over the world. It has a wide variety of uses, but is of particular benefit to the urinary system, reproductive organs, and skin. It is used against hemorrhage and eczema, and a decoction of the root applied locally to the scalp is said to reduce hair loss!
PART USED: whole plant (gathered while in flower)

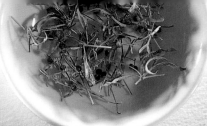

Cleavers
(*Galium aparine*)
Also known as goosegrass, clivers, hayriffe, burweed, or goosebill, cleavers is an excellent tonic for the lymphatic system, and so is used for swollen glands, tonsillitis, and glandular fever (often combined with such herbs as poke root and marigold).

It also benefits the skin, has a long history of use for tumors and ulcers, and may be helpful for painful urinary infections like cystitis.
PART USED: whole plant above ground (gathered before pale green flowers are produced in June and July)

Ginseng
(*Radix ginseng*)
Also known by its Chinese name *Ren Shen*, there are many types of ginseng, each having its own specific properties (sweet, slightly bitter, slightly warm), though all are very strengthening. American ginseng, for example, is cooler in action than Chinese ginseng and therefore more appropriate for use after high fevers. Ginseng is one of the most widely known and valued Chinese herbs (and one of the most expensive!). Traditionally, it has a reputation for increasing fertility and longevity. It is useful in any condition where

Roman chamomile
(*Anthemis nobilis*)
and German chamomile
(*Matricaria chamomilla*)
The actions of both varieties are similar. The name chamomile comes from the Greek word which means "ground apple." It is an excellent mild sedative (suitable for use with children) and reduces inflammation and muscle spasm, such as menstrual cramps. It also aids digestion and reduces flatulence. Used externally, it helps in the healing of wounds and can also be used as a mouthwash for ulcers or gingivitis.
PART USED: flowers (gathered in summer in dry conditions)

there is weakness or exhaustion. In cases of extreme collapse — say, after a serious loss of blood — up to 1 ounce (30g) of ginseng can be decocted and drunk. More commonly, it is used to benefit a weak digestion or aid recovery after a long illness. It also has a calming quality and can be used short-term for palpitations, insomnia, and restlessness accompanied by general debility. *Avoid use in pregnancy, high blood pressure, or where there is no weakness.*
PART USED: root
DOSAGE: 1–9g per day

Lavender
(*Lavandula officinalis*)
This common herb has a variety of uses, based on its cooling and sedative properties: it can be effective for headaches, especially those caused by stress, and is often used in combination with other herbs to deal with depression, nervous exhaustion, and other emotional symptoms. It may aid restful sleep, either taken at bedtime as an infusion or slipped under the pillow in a cheesecloth bag. It is sometimes used for rheumatic pain, especially if this is accompanied by inflammation, and skin rashes.
PART USED: flowers (gathered just

Marigold
(*Calendula officinalis*)
This herb is excellent for external application wherever there are skin rashes, inflammation, or lesions; it speeds the healing process and helps prevent infection of cuts, grazes, and fungal infections. Compresses or poultices work well, and it is also available in homeopathic potency as *Calendula* ointment. Used internally, marigold aids digestion and benefits the gallbladder. It is also a valuable herb for the reproductive system, easing period pains, and regulating the menstrual cycle.
PART USED: flowers or petals (gathered in summer)

Astragalus
(*Radix astragali membranaceus*)
Also known as milk vetch root and by its Chinese name *Huang Qi*, this herb has sweet, slightly warm properties. It is used to strengthen the body, so it helps with fatigue, lack of appetite, and diarrhea. It has the function of "raising the yang *Qi*," so it is useful for prolapses of the uterus, stomach, or rectum. According to Chinese medicine, this drug also "stabilizes the protective *Qi*" and helps strengthen the immune system to guard against frequent colds and illnesses. Today it is used in the treatment of AIDS.
PART USED: root (harvested in spring and fall)
DOSAGE: 9–30g per day

Lemon balm *(below)*
(*Melissa officinalis*)
Also known as balm mint, bee balm, dropsy plant, garden balm, melissa, or sweet balm, this perennial plant is common both wild and cultivated in Europe and parts of the U.S. It is a useful digestive herb, relieving spasm in the intestines and flatulence, and because it also has mild sedative properties, it is helpful for anyone whose digestive problems are associated with anxiety or stress. It benefits the heart and lowers both fever and blood pressure.
PARTS USED: aerial parts (either fresh or dried in the shade)

Elecampane
(*Inula helenium*)
The common name of this herb is said to be a distortion of its Latin title; it is also known as elfwort, scabwort, elfdock, or horseheal. While it is generally cultivated in Britain, the plant grows wild in parts of North America. It soothes coughs, clears catarrh, and has an anti-bacterial action, making it effective for asthma, bronchitis, chest infections, or even emphysema. It has a history of use in tuberculosis, and is good for coughs in children, often combined with such herbs as hyssop and coltsfoot.
PART USED: rhizome (dug up in the fall)

Comfrey
(*Symphytum officinale*)
Also known as knitbone (or nipbone) because of its healing properties in case of fractures, this herb has a long history of external use, too, as a poultice or compress to speed the healing of wounds and lesions. It also works well internally for stomach ulcers and may be beneficial for respiratory infections. *Avoid long-term use.*
PARTS USED: root, rhizome, and leaves

Chinese angelica *(right)*
(*Radix angelicae sinensis*)
Also known by its Chinese names *Dang Gui* and *Tang Kuei*, this beautiful herb with its sweet, acrid, bitter, and warm properties helps to nourish and move the blood, so it is used after childbirth or blood loss, and for anemia and menstrual problems. It is warming, so is helpful in relieving pain that is worse with cold, such as some menstrual cramps and hernia pain. It also moves the bowels, so it is used to treat constipation with dry stools. *Avoid use with diarrhea, bloating, and cases where there are signs of heat* (flushed face, extreme thirst, etc.)
PART USED: root (harvested in the fall)
DOSAGE: 3–15g per day

Passion-flower
(*Passiflora incarnata*)
Also known as maypops
or passion vine, this herb is an
excellent sedative and aids restful
sleep when taken at night. It is also
good for the nerves, and so is used for
neuralgia and herpes zoster (shingles).
Since it releases muscular tension, it
may be useful for asthma or any
condition where the muscles are
in spasm.
    PART USED: dried leaves (gathered
    before flowering)

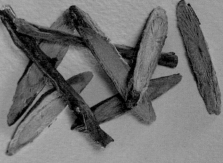

Golden seal *(above)*
(*Hydrastis canadensis*)
Also known as eye root, eye
balm, ground raspberry, and
yellowroot, this plant is a native of
North America and is also a popular
herb in Caribbean cultures. It is a
powerful tonic to the mucous
membranes, resolves phlegm, and
is beneficial to some digestive
disorders including loss of appetite.
It is invaluable in clearing infections
of the upper respiratory tract, but its
prolonged use is not advisable as it is
very drying. For this reason, it is often
added to a prescription in half quantities.
It must be avoided in pregnancy, but can be
useful during labor as it stimulates the
uterine muscles.
PARTS USED: root and rhizome
(unearthed in the fall)

Licorice *(below)*
(*Glycyrrhiza glabra*)
Also known as sweet wood, this plant,
which features in both Western and
Chinese herbalism, benefits the
endocrine system and is therefore
helpful in any illness involving the
adrenal glands. For home use, its
application is more likely to be for
respiratory problems such as
bronchitis, or digestive disorders,
including ulcers, gastritis, and colic.
PART USED: dried root (unearthed in
late fall)

Yarrow
(*Achillea millefolium*)
Also known as milfoil,
nosebleed, and thousand-leaf,
this plant was given its Latin
name by botanists on the basis that it
would have healed the wounds of Achilles, had
he had access to it! This is of course rather
fanciful, but this herb *does* have a valuable
action on wounds, as the Native Americans
have known for many years, using it externally
as a powder on wounds and sores, or infused
to treat burns, fevers, and colds. They also
burn it: the smoke forms an incense to ward
off negative energies. Yarrow is found in the
U.S. and in Europe; the American variety is

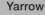

said to be stronger. When taken, it promotes
sweating and so helps the body through
feverish illness; it clears heat from the urinary
tract and so has a role in cystitis; and it is also
said to lower blood pressure.
PART USED: whole plant above ground
(gathered when in flower)

Fennel (left)
(*Foeniculum vulgare*)
Fennel, which appears in both Chinese and Western herbs, relieves flatulence, is good for colic, and improves appetite. It also is said to relieve coughs and improve the flow of milk in women who are breastfeeding. Used externally, as a compress, it relieves inflammation of the eyes (try combining it with eyebright). In both China and the Western world, it is used as a food; but in China, it is also regarded as aiding the digestion and helping pain from hernia.
PART USED: seeds

Elderflower
(*Sambucus nigra*)
Also known as black elder or European elder, all parts can be used medicinally, but in this book reference is only made to the flowers which are collected in spring or summer and dried rapidly. They are useful in the treatment of colds and flu, as they clear catarrh and induce sweating. Hay fever and sinusitis also respond well, and deafness following a cold (usually due to mucus in the Eustachian tubes) may be treated with this herb.
PARTS USED: see above

Thyme
(*Thymus vulgaris*)
Like sage, thyme is a common garden shrub, though it can grow wild; also like sage, it is used for culinary purposes. It does have a broad range of medicinal applications, too – it soothes coughs and sore throats, aids digestion, reduces gas, combats infection, and is mildly astringent so helps in diarrhea and incontinence, especially in children. It is also used for a variety of respiratory problems including whooping cough and bronchitis.
PARTS USED: leaves and flowers (gathered in summer)

Dandelion
(*Taraxacum officinale*)
The name of this common weed is said to come from the French *dents de lion*, meaning lion's teeth – a reflection on the shape of its leaves. It is an excellent diuretic, and a good source of potassium, an essential mineral usually lost from the body when synthetic diuretics are taken. It has a cleansing effect on the liver and gallbladder, so is used in cases of jaundice and indigestion (especially when constipation is involved).
PART USED: root (gathered between June and August) or leaves

Valerian (above)
(*Valeriana officinalis*)
Also called Capon's tail, this herb is an outstanding nervine relaxant, combining well with other herbs such as hops and passion-flower to deal with insomnia in adults. It also reduces muscle cramp and is therefore effective against pain caused by spasm, such as colic or menstrual cramps. It is an excellent sedative and may be used instead of chemical tranquillizers if the patient is tense, anxious, or panicky. It is not recommended for long-term use, however; after taking it for about six weeks, have a three-week break before using it again.
PARTS USED: root and rhizome (unearthed in autumn)

Chrysanthemum flower
(*Chrysanthemi morifolium*)
Also known by its Chinese name *Ju Hua*, this flower has sweet, bitter, and slightly cold properties. It is most commonly used for clearing colds accompanied by fever and headache. It can also be used on its own to help strengthen the eyes, for conditions such

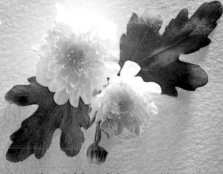

Coltsfoot (*above*)
(*Tussilago farfara*)
Also known as coughwort, horsehoof, British tobacco, butterbur, or foal's-foot, this herb with its hoof-shaped leaves has a legendary effect on coughs and most other respiratory problems, including asthma, bronchitis, emphysema, and whooping cough. It is soothing, antispasmodic, and expectorant, and combines well with hyssop, elecampane, lobelia, and other herbs which benefit the lungs.
PARTS USED: leaves (gathered in May or June) and flowers (usually picked in March or April before they have fully bloomed)

as red, painful, and dry eyes, blurred vision, and spots in front of the eyes. It has a calming effect and can help with dizziness and headaches caused by tension.
PART USED: flowers (harvested in full bloom)
DOSAGE: 4–15g per day

Vervain
(*Verbena officinalis*)
This herb is an excellent mild sedative, which strengthens the nervous system while also having a calming effect. It is available in teabags in parts of Europe and makes a pleasant bedtime drink. This herb also helps deal with depression, especially if this is caused by the depletion of energy after a virus, and is often most effective combined with oats and skullcap. It benefits the liver and gallbladder, (organs which Chinese medicine see as playing a role in depression), and so may be of help in jaundice and hepatitis
PART USED: whole plant above ground (gathered in July just before blooming)

Sage
(*Salvia officinalis*)
Also known as red sage or garden sage, this herb has a specific action on the mouth and throat, and will benefit most conditions in that area, especially where there is inflammation. It is often used as a mouthwash or gargle, and will benefit sore throats, mouth ulcers, bleeding gums, tonsillitis, and laryngitis. It will also work for these conditions when taken internally, and its other actions include reducing flatulence, slowing the production of breast milk, and inducing sweating. It has another use in the Native American tradition: the dried leaves are burned, and the smoke is used as incense for cleansing negative energies – white mountain sage is preferred for this use. *It should be avoided in pregnancy.*
PART USED: leaves (gathered in May or June, and dried in the shade)

OTHER HERBS

This section briefly describes all the remaining herbs mentioned in the *Ailments* section, so that you can check their suitability before taking or prescribing them. Many herbals list a thousand herbs or more; this book includes only about a hundred, which may still sound a lot if you are new to the subject! There is no need to attempt to familiarize yourself with all of them; in time you will get to know the ones you use often. Here we have simply listed each herb's common name, Latin name, and main actions.

Borage
(*Borago officinalis*)

Agnus castus berries
(*Vitex agnus-castus*)
Also called chaste tree; tonic and normalizer for the female reproductive system.

Agrimony   (*Agrimonia eupatoria*)
Has an astringent action on the digestive tract; specific for diarrhea in children.

Barley grain   (*Hordeum vulgare*)
Cooling and moist, benefiting the stomach, throat, and bladder; commonly used for cystitis.

Basil   (*Ocimum basilicum*)
Used against stomach cramps, vomiting, constipation, and gastroenteritis.

Bayberry   (*Myrica cerifera*)
A circulatory stimulant; valuable in diarrhea, colitis, sore throats, and colds.

Black cohosh   (*Cimicifuga racemosa*)
Native American herb, excellent to relax and normalize the reproductive system.

Blackcurrant leaves   (*Ribes nigrum*)
Cool and drying action; helpful to the digestive and urinary systems.

Blue cohosh
(*Caulophyllum thalictroides*)
Also called squaw root and papoose root; uterine tonic; helps delayed periods or labor pains.

Boneset   (*Eupatorium perfoliatum*)
Excellent remedy for flu, colds, and fevers.

Borage leaves   (*Borago officinalis*)
Benefit the adrenal gland; help in stress, fevers, and convalescence.

Buchu   (*Agathosma betulina*)
Diuretic, very useful for urinary infections or whenever there is pain or discomfort on urination.

Burdock root   (*Arctium lappa*)
Valuable for dry skin conditions, rheumatism, kidney problems, and wounds.

Caraway seeds   (*Carum carvil*)
Benefit the digestion, helping flatulence and colic and loss of appetite or diarrhea.

Cardamom   (*Elettaria cardamomum*)
Reduces gas and griping pains; improves appetite and flow of saliva.

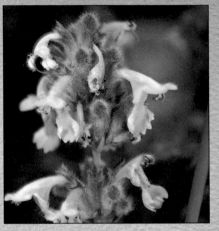

Catnip   (*Nepeta cataria*)
Eases stomach upsets involving flatulence; also good for colds and flu.

Cayenne   (*Capsicum minimum*)
Stimulant to the digestive and circulatory systems; antiseptic.

Celery seeds   (*Apium graveolens*)
Diuretic with specific action on arthritis, rheumatism, and other joint pains.

Chickweed   (*Stellaria media*)
Cool moist herb used externally for wounds or rashes, internally for rheumatism.

Cinnamon   (*Cinnamomum zeylanicum*)
Helps against gas, nausea, vomiting, and diarrhea.

Cloves   (*Eugenia caryophyllus*)
Stimulates digestion, alleviates nausea, vomiting and flatulence; antiseptic and anesthetic properties make it useful locally, e.g., for toothache.

Cornsilk (*Zea mays*)
Cool moist herb which soothes any inflammation of the urinary tract.

Couchgrass (*Agropyron repens*)
Also benefits the urinary system; used for cystitis, urethritis, prostatitis, and kidney stones.

Crampbark (*Vinurnum opulus*)
Named after its action, relaxes muscle tension anywhere in the body; may prevent threatened miscarriage.

Damiana (*Turnera aphrodisiaca*)
Tonic for hormonal and nervous systems, and antidepressant.

Eyebright (*Euphrasia officinalis*)
As its name suggests, reduces inflammation in the eyes; also benefits the mucous membranes and clears catarrh.

False unicorn root
(*Chamaelirium luteum*)
Tonic for both male and female reproductive systems; used in ovarian pain, threatened miscarriage, and late or absent menstruation.

Feverfew (*Tanacetum parthenium*)
Relieves migraines and headaches, "hot" arthritis, dizziness, tinnitus, and painful or hesitant menstrual flow.

Forsythia (*Forsythia*)
Also known by its Chinese name *Lian Qiao*. Expels "wind-heat," i.e., sudden onset of feverish virus; therefore used at first sign of cold or flu.

Ginger (*Zingiber officinale*)
Stimulates the circulation, induces sweating, settles flatulence, and relieves sore throats.

Hawthorn berries
(*Crataegus oxyacanthoides*)
Normalize the activity of the heart, and therefore useful in palpitations and high blood pressure.

Honeysuckle (*Lonicera*)
Also known by its Chinese name *Jin Yin Hua*. Often used in combination with forsythia in a slightly higher dosage (9–15g, daily) for feverish colds and flu.

Hops (*Humulus lupulus*)
Sedative herb, relieving anxiety, insomnia, and nervous diarrhea or indigestion. *Avoid long-term use; do not prescribe if patient is depressed.*

Hyssop (*Hyssopus officinalis*)
Excellent to soothe coughs, induce sweating, and calm anxiety states.

Jamaican dogwood
(*Piscidia erythrina*)
Acts as a pain reliever and sedative; particularly useful if there is insomnia as a result of pain.

Lime blossom (*Tilia europea*)
A relaxant herb which lowers blood pressure; also used against migraines and colds.

Longan fruit
Also known by its Chinese name *Long Yan Rou*. Nourishes the blood and calms the spirit; used for insomnia, forgetfulness, palpitations, and dizziness.

Marjoram (*Origanum vulgare*)
This culinary herb has a valuable action in colds, coughs, and flu, as it induces sweating and has antiseptic properties.

Marshmallow (*Althaea officinalis*)
Both root and leaf are cool and moist; the root acts on the digestion and skin, the leaf on the lungs and urinary system.

Meadowsweet (*Filipendula ulmaria*)
Excellent digestive remedy; used to treat childhood diarrhea and also rheumatism.

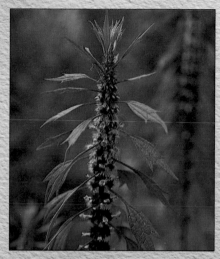

Motherwort (*Leonurus cardiaca*)
Benefits circulation, therefore useful in heart conditions and to regularize menstruation; often used in menopause.

Mullein (*Verbascum thapsus*)
Has an anti-inflammatory effect on the lungs, and so soothes coughs. The oil is used to soften ear wax.

Oats (*Avena sativa*)
Nourishing to the nervous system; excellent for nervous exhaustion and depression.

Parsley (*Petroselinum crispum*)
Besides being rich in Vitamin C, is a diuretic, can help bring on menstruation, and eases gas. *Avoid large amounts in pregnancy.*

Pasque flower (*Anemone pulsatilla*)
Relieves period pains and tension headaches; also useful for the skin and respiratory system.

Pennyroyal
(*Mentha pulegium*)
Releases muscle spasms, relieving colicky indigestion. Its main use is to bring on delayed menstruation. *Avoid in pregnancy.*

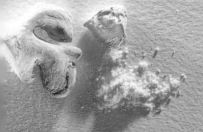

Peppermint
(*Mentha piperata*)
Rich in volatile oils, is an excellent digestive, relieving flatulence, nausea, and morning sickness; also helps reduce feverish colds and flu.

Prickly ash
(*Xanthoxylum americanum*)
Stimulates circulation and lymphatic drainage; used in rheumatism and skin diseases.

Raspberry leaf
(*Rubus idaeus*)
Traditionally used to strengthen and tone the uterine muscles during pregnancy and labor; also valuable for diarrhea and mouth ulcers.

Red clover
(*Trifolium pratense*)
Most commonly used for skin problems in children; also against coughs.

Rhubarb root   (*Rheum palmatum*)
Not the same as garden rhubarb; excellent for constipation and cleansing the intestines.

Roses
(*Rosa gallica*)
Any red rose petals can be used medicinally, usually hybrid perpetuals; also the hips of the dog rose have similar actions: as a tonic or astringent, or to calm the nerves and boost immunity.

Rosemary
(*Rosmarinus officinalis*)
Acts as a stimulant to the circulation and nervous system; helps digestion and muscular pain.

Rue   (*Ruta graveolens*)
Regulates menses and eases spasm in the digestive tract.
Avoid in pregnancy.

Saw palmetto   (*Serenoa serrulata*)
Strengthens the male reproductive system and is beneficial in prostatitis and urinary infections.

Shepherd's purse
(*Capsella bursa-pastoris*)
Has a mild diuretic action, also regulates menstruation; its astringent effect helps against diarrhea and bleeding.

Skullcap   (*Scutellaria laterifolia*)
Nervine tonic and relaxant: excellent for premenstrual and other tension.

Slippery elm   (*Ulmus fulva*)
Has a cool moist action on inflamed or sensitive digestive systems; good during convalescence.

Squaw vine   (*Mitchella repens*)
Native American herb, excellent in preparation for childbirth; also helps period pains.

St. John's wort   (*Hypericum perforatum*)
Sedative and analgesic, therefore useful in many painful conditions; also helps menopausal mood swings.

Tangerine peel
Also known by its Chinese name *Chen Pi*. Benefits digestion, relieves nausea, settles flatulence, and bloating.

Tansy   (*Tanacetum vulgare*)
Clears intestinal worms from the digestive tract, improves digestion, and brings on menstruation.
Avoid use long-term or in pregnancy.

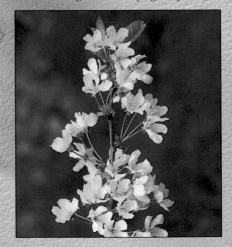

Wild cherry   (*Prunus serotina*)
Soothes the cough reflex, useful in any form of cough.

Wild yam   (*Dioscorea villosa*)
Benefits digestion and menstruation; relieves painful, inflamed joints and regulates hormonal function.

Yellow dock   (*Rumex crispus*)
Cleanses the blood, good for chronic skin conditions, and eases constipation.

CHINESE HERBAL FORMULAE

These combinations of Chinese herbs are based on well-known traditional herbal prescriptions. They are made into pill form, a more convenient way to take herbs than decoctions which require daily cooking and drinking. They are less potent than decoctions but still very effective.

Western manufacturers are now producing variations on these traditional formulae. Pills or powders may include other herbs which enhance or slightly alter their actions. The brand name will be different, but the name of the traditional formulae on which they are based should be stated.

Bi Yan Pian "Clear the nose pill"
Helps clear heat and congestion in hay fever, rhinitis, and sinus problems.
DOSAGE: 4–6 tablets, three times daily.

Dang Gui Bu Xue Tang "Angelica decoction to tonify the blood"
Nourishes the blood and *Qi*; often used after childbirth or with anemia.
DOSAGE: 5 tablets, two or three times daily.

Nu Ke Ba Zhen Wan "Women's precious pills"
Very good general tonic for women, especially after childbirth, fatigue, or blood loss.
DOSAGE: 5 tablets, two or three times daily.

Qi Ju Di Huang Wan Lycium fruit, chrysanthemum, and rehmannia pill
This nourishing formula is used for dry or painful eyes with loss of visual acuity, photophobia, and tearing when exposed to the wind. Helpful for the elderly.

Shen Ling Bai Zhu Pian
Benefits digestion, especially with loose stools and diarrhea; good for gas, bloating, indigestion. Safe for children and long-term use.
DOSAGE: 5 tablets, twice daily (halve for children).

Si Jun Zi Tang "Four gentlemen decoction"
This gentle formula may be taken over a period of time to strengthen the digestion and *Qi* (vital force), for example after a debilitating illness.
DOSAGE: 5 tablets, two or three times daily.

Tian Wang Bu Xin Wan "Emperor's tea"
Calming formula, used for insomnia, anxiety, and palpitations.
DOSAGE: 5 pills, twice daily.

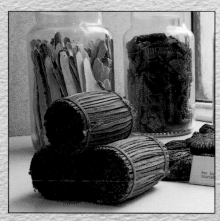

Chinese medicinal herbs are taken as decoctions or ground into pills and powders.

Xiao Yao Wan "Free and easy wanderer"
Benefits the liver and circulation, thus helping a range of symptoms including digestive and menstrual problems.
DOSAGE: 5 pills, twice daily.

Xiang Sha Liu Jun Wan "Six gentlemen tea pill"
Strengthens weak digestion; helps with bloating and flatulence.
DOSAGE: 5 pills, twice daily.

Yin Qiao Jie Du Pien "Dispell heat tablets"
Used immediately at the first sign of a feverish cold or flu, will help sore throats and sometimes prevent the virus from developing.
DOSAGE: 5 pills every 2–3 hours on first day, reducing.

Yu Ping Feng San "Jade windscreen powder"
Used to protect against recurrent colds and strengthen immunity; can be taken over a period of several months.
DOSAGE: 5 tablets, two or three times daily.

BASIC PRINCIPLES

Herbs are available from suppliers in a number of different forms, the main ones being loose dried herbs and tinctures. It is largely a matter of personal preference which one you choose; some people enjoy handling the loose herbs, and consider their texture, appearance, and aroma essential to their healing properties. On the other hand, there is no doubt that tinctures (a solution of the herb in alcohol) are more convenient and keep longer. Feel free to experiment until you find the form that suits you. There are a few guidelines, however. Some herbs – golden seal, yarrow, and valerian, for example – have a taste which most people find unpleasant, and therefore if the prescription you are making up contains one of these, you may find tinctures more palatable; as tinctures are so concentrated, they are taken in smaller quantities. Herbs which consist of the root or bark of the plant, such as echinacea, will need boiling (known as decoction) for the full therapeutic action to be derived.

Because tinctures consist of the herb suspended in an alcoholic base, and the energy of alcohol tends to be heating, some herbalists prefer to avoid tinctures for certain conditions, such as fevers or inflammation. To avoid this problem, take them well-diluted.

It is possible to make your own herbal tea bags from small cloth bags to avoid having to strain an infusion.

PRECAUTIONS

Herbs are generally safe to use for old and young, with very few side effects. However, caution is necessary in some conditions, such as pregnancy. In pregnant women a great deal of energy is being invested in creating new life; this amazing system is a delicate balance which functions best with minimal intervention. There are a number of herbs which can enhance a woman's health in pregnancy; but there are also some which are unsuitable and must be avoided. A full list is given in the section on pregnancy (page 43).

Some sensitive individuals may have an adverse reaction to certain herbs. If this happens, in the form of rashes, headaches, nausea, or any other unfamiliar symptoms, it is advisable to stop taking the herbs and consult a qualified herbalist. People with weak digestion occasionally have difficulty tolerating tinctures; if they upset your stomach, try taking the herbs as an infusion or decoction instead.

CHOOSING THE HERBS

Herbs work holistically; they have a range of actions that work harmoniously together on the human organism, which is one of their advantages over allopathic drugs, which generally have a single, fairly aggressive, action. For this reason, it is usually quite safe to take just one herb. For example, if you are getting flu, you may want to take echinacea; it will support your immune system, help combat the virus, and reduce excessive mucus.

However, it may be helpful to take two or more herbs together to cover a broader range of actions. For example, you may want to combine echinacea with two or three other herbs, such as yarrow to help with a fever; cleavers or marigold for swollen glands; and golden seal to clear the mucous membranes. If you are restless or having difficulty sleeping, you can add a relaxing herb such as skullcap or passion-flower. Most of the herbal prescriptions suggested in this book consist of several herbs which combine well together. You can work out your own prescriptions when you become familiar with the herbs. It is also useful to remember that herbs work on an emotional as well as a physical level; so, if you are choosing a herb for a cough, and the patient is also excitable or insomniac, you may want to choose hyssop which has mild sedative qualities as well as being an expectorant.

The Bach flower remedies are a complete system which uses the healing properties of flowers, prescribed solely according to the patient's emotional state. They are on pages 56–9.

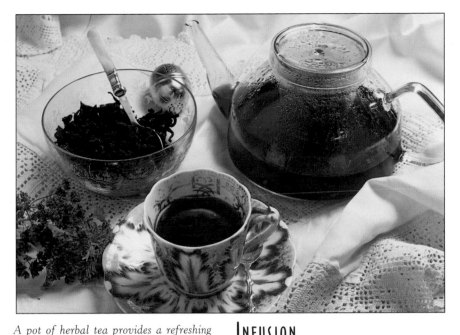

A pot of herbal tea provides a refreshing alternative to black tea or coffee, offering a pleasant drink and a remedy for your ailment.

INFUSION

An infusion is like a tea of herb or herbal mixture – in fact, most people use a teapot to prepare their infusions. Infusion is a good method for preparing leaves and flowers, such as marshmallow, lavender, or nettles. While most infusions require steeping the leaves in hot water, if your mixture contains any roots or bark, you will have to boil it first.

To make an infusion, put 2 tsp of the herbal mixture in a warmed teapot (a glass or china teapot is best for this, avoid metal if possible) and add two cupfuls of boiling water. Leave to steep for 10–15 minutes, stirring occasionally. It is usual to drink the infusion hot, but there is no reason why you should not take it cold or even iced, if you prefer; if you need to sweeten the tea, use honey, barley malt, apple juice concentrate or liquorice root.

RECOMMENDED DOSAGES

	ADULTS	CHILDREN AND 70+
INFUSIONS:	1–2 cups, three times daily	½ cup, three times daily
DECOCTIONS:	1 cup, two or three times daily	½ cup, three times daily
TINCTURES:	10 drops – 5ml (1 tbsp), three times daily	5–10 drops, three times daily

The quantities shown in this easy-reference table will be similar whether you are taking a single herb or a mixture. Where a combination of herbs is recommended, it is generally appropriate to mix them in equal quantities. Some herbs may appear in half quantities compared with the other herbs in the prescription; golden seal is one such herb, as it has a slightly aggressive drying action and is best taken in small quantities for short periods of time. However, the above dosages are generally applicable and, where they vary from this, they have been explained elsewhere, such as Chinese herbs where the exact weight in grams should be decocted for longer than usual (45 minutes).

DECOCTION

This means boiling or simmering. It is the method used for any herb which consists of a woody or hard part of the plant: roots, bark, seeds, or rhizomes. Add about 1 oz. (30g) of the herbal mixture to each 6 oz. (500ml) of water in a pan. It is best to use a pan made of glass or ceramic. It's okay to use a metal pan if that's all you have, but avoid aluminum at all costs, as it is toxic and traces will leach into the herbs. Bring to a boil and simmer for 10–15 minutes, then let the mixture cool for a short time and strain it, squeezing the herbs to

Simmer roots, barks, and seeds gently for 10–15 minutes to extract their essences and make a beneficial medicinal tea.

extract all the beneficial juices.

One disadvantage of decoction is that it may tend to boil off the volatile oils in some plants, thus losing their remedial effect: for example, the volatile oils in fennel, aniseed, and peppermint benefit digestion, and so these herbs will not be so effective if boiled. If you have a prescription which contains roots and leaves, you may prefer to prepare them separately and then mix the resulting liquids before drinking them; or, after making the decoction, add the leaves and flowers while the mixture is still hot, and leave the brew to stand for 10 minutes. Alternatively, roots *can* be effectively infused if they are finely powdered beforehand; some herbalists now stock powdered herbs.

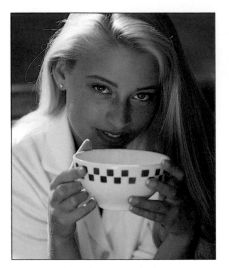

Drinking herbal teas regularly over a period of time can enhance health, increase vitality, and induce a general feeling of wellbeing.

CHINESE HERBS

Chinese herbs are generally boiled for longer – about 45 minutes is usual. The result is quite dense and may taste unpleasant, but is generally very effective!

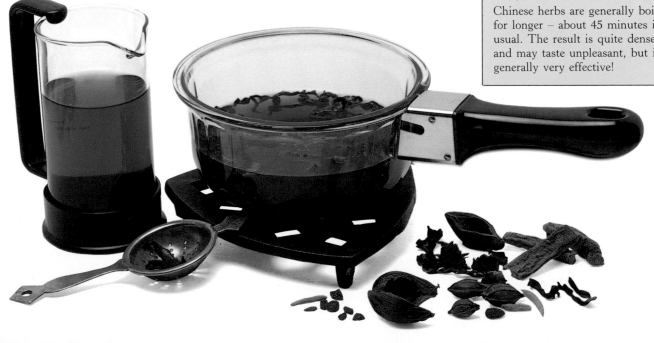

TINCTURES

This term generally refers to a herbal solution in alcohol; more rarely, it can be used for a preparation based in vinegar or glycerin. The advantages of tinctures include their very long shelf life (about two years), convenience, and the fact that alcohol acts as a good solvent for most of the active ingredients of the herb. Tinctures may be somewhat more expensive than loose herbs in their dried form.

It is possible to make tinctures at home, but it is a lengthy process and the result will probably not be as strong or last as well as those bought from a herbal supplier. Such suppliers often sell the tinctures in 1 pint (500ml) bottles, which is a fairly large amount for the home user; some will sell them in smaller quantities however, or even mix up a number of herbs in one bottle, if that suits your purpose.

Many people dilute tinctures in half a glass of water or apple juice, though you can dilute them in a cup of tea! Coffee itself has strong actions as a diuretic and stimulant, so it would not serve well as a dilutant. Since alcohol boils off at very low temperatures, an added benefit of the tea is that some of the alcohol in the tincture will evaporate. For children, the dose is shown in the table on page 19. Take at least half an hour before meals.

TONIC WINES

It is also possible to steep herbs in wine to produce your own tonic wines: they are said to taste very pleasant although they will not last as long as an alcohol-based tincture. Many aperitifs and liqueurs started out as herbal remedies intended to aid digestion.

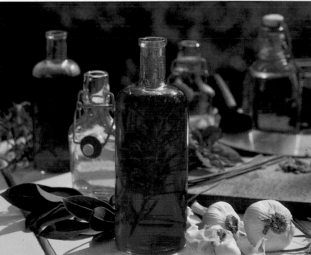

Herbal tinctures are easy to take and last for up to two years.

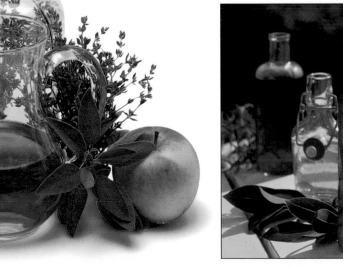

Alcohol and vinegar are used to preserve herbs.

SYRUPS

These may be a useful way to persuade children to take herbs – they are also soothing in the case of coughs. Frequent use is not really recommended because of the harmful effects of too much sugar; you are in danger of cancelling out the benefit of the herbs!

Syrups are simple to make: combine 1¼ pints (600ml) of boiling water with 2 lbs (900g) of sugar in a pan, bring back to a boil, stirring continuously, and immediately turn off the heat. Mix the resulting syrup base with the required tincture/s (three parts syrup to one part tincture) and store in the refrigerator. Syrups also work well used as a gargle.

Coltsfoot syrup helps to soothe and stop coughs.

Children find syrups are a pleasant way of taking herbs.

TABLETS AND POWDERS

Some herbs are readily available in tablet form: echinacea tablets, for example, are often found in health-food stores, as are a range of herbal sedative tablets, usually combining valerian, passion-flower, hops, and extract of lettuce.

Chinese herbal patent formulae – tried and tested prescriptions, some of which have been in use for thousands of years – are also most commonly found in tablet form (see pages 26–7). They are sometimes also available in tincture form.

Powdered herbs are becoming more available, and these can be eaten dry, mixed with water and drunk, or put in gelatin capsules and swallowed. The variety which are freeze-dried from a decoction are best; if they are simply a finely ground version of the dried herb, it is unlikely that the full medicinal value of the herb is obtained.

Passion-flower is a common ingredient of herbal tablets to aid sleep and relaxation.

COMPRESSES AND POULTICES

These are two more methods of applying herbal remedies externally. Compresses consist of any clean cloth or absorbent cotton soaked in a hot infusion or decoction and applied to the skin, as hot as is comfortable.

Poultices consist of a paste made by mixing the herbs with water; this is then placed between layers of thin cloth such as gauze or cheesecloth. Applied locally, they can speed the healing process in affected areas; herbs such as comfrey or marsh mallow are often used.

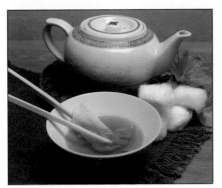

Compress – *Soak a clean cloth in an appropriate herbal tea. Use to heal external injuries or skin conditions.*

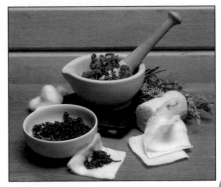

Comfrey poultice – *Leaves are used externally to heal sprains and severe cuts, soothe pain and inflammation, and drain boils and abscesses.*

BATHS

The healing properties of herbs are absorbed very efficiently through the skin, so herbal baths (either the whole body or a foot or hand bath) deserve a mention. For a whole-body bath, either add about 1 pint (500ml) of a decoction or infusion to the water, or hang the fresh or dried herbs in a gauze bag under the hot faucet while running the water.

Foot baths and hand baths consist of the undiluted herbal preparation. This is an effective method to induce a good night's sleep; use valerian, skullcap, and hops for adults, or lime blossom and chamomile, which have a gentler action, for children. Similarly, some infusions, when cool, are excellent for local external application: a weak infusion of eyebright, for

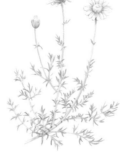

Chamomile
(Anthemis nobilis)

example, works very well for bathing sore or infected eyes. This method is effective for animals, too (Remember to allow the liquid to cool first!)

Using herbs in baths is a simple way of relaxing.

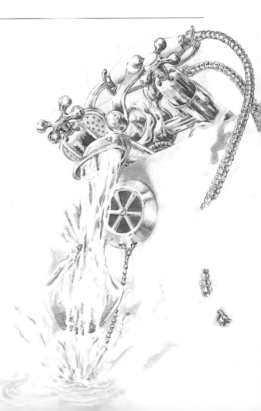

YIN AND YANG

The theory of yin and yang is attributable to early Chinese civilization and its philosophers. It is quite possible to use and prescribe herbs without a thorough understanding of these principles, but it is an important part of Chinese herbal medicine and has a bearing on the understanding of some Western herbal actions, too.

The yin-yang theory postulates the idea that all the systems in the universe consist of these two conflicting yet interdependent energies: from yin and yang originate all the myriad forms of creation. They can be roughly likened to water and fire in their respective natures, but there is a risk of over-simplifying these concepts to make them comprehensible to the Western mind! The following list may give you an idea of the ways in which these two forces exist in contrast to each other:

From these comparisons, it is hopefully becoming evident that the nature of yang tends to be hot, bright, upward, and active; it is often seen as embodying a more masculine energy. Yin, on the other hand, is cool, moist, inward, and more nourishing, and is generally seen as being more feminine in its nature. There are no value judgments in this system; each energy provides a perfect complement and antithesis to the other, and cannot exist in isolation.

Ideally, these energies should be in balance in the human body/mind; if they are, good health will prevail. If either energy is depleted, it will affect the other adversely, and illness will eventually be the result. This interdependence is demonstrated sometimes in terms of disease; when suffering from a feverish illness accompanied by a high temperature and sweating, for example, the person feels hot, dry, and lacking in energy, and this feeling can sometimes last for a time after the fever has passed. This

YIN
Marsh mallow leaves
(Althaea officinalis)

YIN (WATER)	YANG (FIRE)
cold	heat
moon	sun
below	above
heavy	light
dim	bright
still	active
being	doing
wet	dry
slow	rapid
night	day

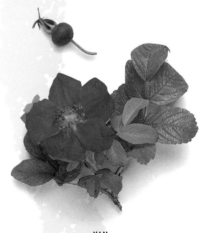

YIN
Rose
(Rosa gallica officinalis)

is because the body fluids (yin) have been depleted by the heating effect of the fever. Herbs can help to restore the water/fire balance in the body.

Some herbs are more cool and moist (or yin) in their energy and actions, and they can be used to cool, lubricate, and soften the digestive tract or lungs. Examples are marsh mallow, coltsfoot, and slippery elm. Others are more drying and warming, such as lady's mantle, which is a tonic for the reproductive system, and is more yang in its action. Some herbs are both cooling *and* drying: golden seal and echinacea are good examples, which is why they are so useful for clearing infections in all parts of the body.

In general, the leaves and flowers of a plant are more cooling in action, and its roots more warming, though there are exceptions to this rule. When choosing herbs for a particular individual or symptom, it is helpful to have an awareness of the "temperature" of the herbs you are using, in relation to the energy of the patient. This is particularly true when using Chinese herbs and patent formulas, which can be quite powerful (see page 17).

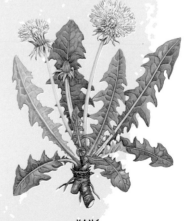

YANG
Root ginger
(Zingiber officinale)

YANG
Cinnamon
(Cinnamomum zeylanicum)

YANG
Dandelion root
(Taraxacum officinale)

CHINESE HERBAL MEDICINE

Chinese herbal medicine has a rich tradition that dates back to manuscripts from the end of the third century B.C. found in the Ma Wang Tui tomb in the Hunan province. The Yellow Emperor's Inner Classic, believed to have been compiled about 2,000 years ago, contains many of the theoretical foundations of traditional Chinese medicine. The true originator of Chinese herbal formulae is Zhang Zhong-Jing, who wrote his treatise, the *Shang han za bing lun* (Discussion of Cold-induced Disorders and Miscellaneous Diseases) at the end of the third century A.D. These basic formulas have evolved over the years to play a large part in modern Chinese medicine.

The other major work, the *Wen bing tiao bian* (Systematic Differentiation of Warm Diseases), written in the late eighteenth century by Wu Ju-Tong, provides further insight into the diagnoses and treatments using Chinese herbal formulas. These classical texts have been the basis for much debate that has led to the development of many of the formulas that are used in modern Chinese medicine.

The properties of Chinese herbs were discovered long before modern scientific methods were developed. Centuries of testing through trial and error, as well as the discussions that the many treatises on herbs have engendered, have led to well-defined descriptions of the herbs. More recently, the herbs have been put through the scrutiny of biochemical analysis. In some cases, this has confirmed their traditional uses. In others, researchers have been puzzled as to why certain herbal combinations actually cure disease. New uses have also been discovered for some herbs – for example, some have been found to be anticarcinogenic.

Traditionally, Chinese herbs have been classified according to the "temperature" they induce, their taste, the "channel" they enter, and whether they are yin, yang, or neutral. For example, astragalus (*Huang Qi*) is sweet and slightly warming, enters the lung and spleen channels, and is strengthening to the yang *Qi*. As mentioned in the section on yin and yang (pages 24–5), the nature of yang tends to be hot, bright, upward, and active. One of the uses of astragalus is for the treatment of prolapses, to help raise the descending energy which is

A Chinese herbal prescription can contain a striking variety of herbs.

pulling the organ downward. Its sweet taste means that it is strengthening and nourishing. By entering the lung and spleen channels, it is very helpful in enhancing the immune system and preventing illness.

It is more common to use several Chinese herbs in combination than it is to use them individually. Chinese herbal formulas combine different herbs that work together effectively and in balance. One of the favorite ways of understanding prescriptions was based on the political structure of the Chinese dynasty. The name of the Chinese formulas known as the four gentlemen decoction (*Si Jun Zi Tang*) was derived from the Confucian term for a person whose behavior is exemplary, and the number four, which is considered harmonious. It is a simple, moderate prescription of four herbs used to strengthen digestion and tonify *Qi*. The chief herb, also known as the "emperor" or *Jun* herb, is ginseng (*Ren Shen*), which is a powerful tonic for the digestion and overall energy. The "minister" or *Chen* herb – white *Atractylodes* rhizome (*Bai Zhu*) – acts as the adviser. These two herbs work synergistically to improve the digestive function. The "assistant" or *Zuo* herb is poria (*Fu Ling*) which is for strengthening and drying, and prevents the prescription from becoming too cloying and bloating. It combines well with the "envoy" or *Shi* herb, honey-fried licorice (*Zhi Gan Cao*) whose function it is to deliver the whole prescription to the digestive tract.

Chinese Patent Remedies are classical prescriptions made into pill form. This is a more

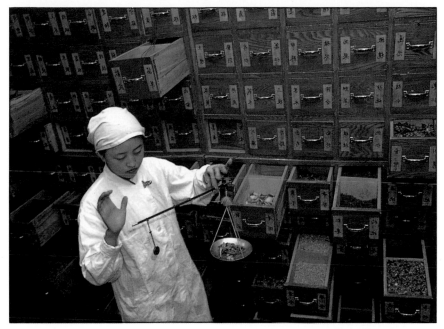

For centuries, the Chinese have practiced herbal medicine, providing many cures which have been adapted to treat modern illnesses.

Chinese herbal formulas are a combination of herbs which work together in a balanced and harmonious way.

convenient way to take the herbs, though generally they are not as strong as those prepared as decoctions. Different herbal companies produce variations on these prescriptions which will be called by other names, but the original formula should be stated. Many modern herbal companies are attempting to expand on the traditional formulas to focus their actions on long-term illnesses, especially AIDS and cancer. Hopefully with these new insights into the wisdom of the past, more successful treatments, or better still, ways of preventing these illnesses from taking hold in the first place, will be found.

SPECIFIC APPLICATIONS

Herbs form part of the spectrum of natural or energetic medicine, and as such, like all holistic methods, they are best used preventatively. For example, by treating a cold or flu in its early stages, you should be able to prevent a chest infection or bronchitis; similarly, tackling the symptoms of indigestion early may deter the development of a peptic ulcer. Most people feel happier and more whole when they are taking responsibility for their own health and have some control over what they put into their bodies, and quite often the judicious use of herbs can prevent a visit to the doctor altogether. However, when the symptoms are serious or intractable, seeking professional advice is then obviously a sensible course of action.

Where appropriate in this section, other areas of complementary medicine that have been found helpful for specific complaints are mentioned, and of course everyone should use their own judgment as to when to consult a doctor. There is no doubt that modern medicine saves lives, and drugs such as antibiotics have a valuable place in the case of severe infection; however, their indiscriminate use is harmful to the digestive tract and the immune system. If you do use allopathic medicine, herbs may be very successful in alleviating any side effects or unpleasant consequences.

Evening primrose
(*Oenothera biennis*)

This section is arranged in order of the systems of the body:

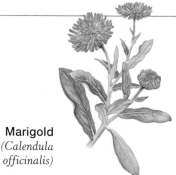

Marigold
(Calendula officinalis)

THE HEAD AND CHEST

pages 30 – 35
This first section looks at common viral conditions affecting the respiratory tract, such as coughs and colds, sore throats, and influenza. Herbs for more chronic problems such as migraine, heachache, and rhinitis (hay fever) are also discussed.

RECOMMENDED HERBS

After finding the herbs recommended for a particular problem, you should then cross-check in the section on the herbs and their actions (pages 8–17), to make sure that they are suitable for you and your symptoms.

THE DIGESTIVE SYSTEM

pages 36 – 39
Herbal medicine can be extremely useful for dealing with discomfort of the digestive tract. This section deals with a variety of problems including heartburn, nausea, diarrhea, constipation, and irritable bowel syndrome.

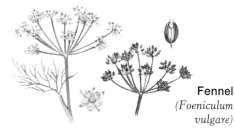

Fennel
(Foeniculum vulgare)

EMOTIONS

pages 52 – 55
Anyone can be affected by stress, anxiety, or sleeplessness at various times in their lives. Herbs cannot eliminate the problems you face, but may enable you to deal with them

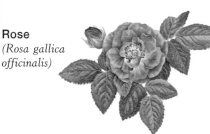

Rose
(Rosa gallica officinalis)

THE REPRODUCTIVE AND URINARY SYSTEMS

pages 40 – 45
You can use herbs to facilitate smoother functioning of the reproductive organs, helping to make the important times of transition in women's lives – puberty, childbirth, and menopause – more positive events.

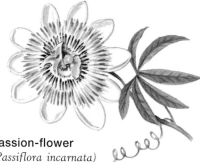

Passion-flower
(Passiflora incarnata)

WHOLE BODY AND SKIN

pages 46 – 51
This section deals with complaints which can affect all or part of the body: painful conditions, rashes, and tiredness. This includes herbs for problems such as arthritis, rheumatism, post-viral fatigue, eczema, and acne.

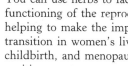

Licorice
(Glycyrrhiza glabra)

more easily. A number of herbs are included which are calming, facilitate sleep, or alleviate depression. However, we recommend you to consult your doctor, counselor, or therapist if your emotional problems persist.

HEAD AND CHEST

Illnesses that affect the head and the chest are the very common conditions that usually people get at least once a year. The Chinese would say that the head and neck, being at the top of the body and often the most exposed to cold winds and wet weather, are where disease first enters the body. In the West, it is accepted that viruses travel through the air, so it is often in the respiratory system that they take hold.

A few simple herbs can give much relief without the need for other medication, especially if they are taken early. Many people find that herbs are the most effective way of treating catarrhal conditions – far better than antibiotics. Of course, if you have a high fever, pain, or a condition which is not clearing, you must seek professional medical advice. If you do need to take antibiotics, it is fine to continue to take the herbs listed.

COMMON COLD

Colds are often seen as a nuisance. Actually, they are your body's way of saying it is tired and needs a break. A cold is a good time for the body to thoroughly clear out all the toxins that have accumulated through daily life. These processes can be helped by resting, drinking lots of liquids and eating lightly, and taking vitamin C and herbs.

Peppermint
(Mentha piperata)

Yarrow
(Achillea millefolium)

ELDERFLOWER, PEPPERMINT, AND YARROW

These herbs are aromatic and drying; very useful for the early stage of a cold. Drink decoctions as hot as possible, every few hours. They will help to clear your head and dry up your runny nose.

BONESET AND NEPETA

These herbs help to clear mild fevers and to ease the aches and pains of flu. Combine with other herbs as needed. Generally, a fever with sweating is a good way of getting rid of a cold, and these herbs will promote perspiration. This will then cause the fever to "break," and the temperature will start to go down.

Honeysuckle
(Lonicera)

Yin Qiao Jie Du Pien
This Chinese patent remedy has an excellent reputation for getting rid of colds. It has to be taken at the first signs of a cold, before it is established. Take 5 pills every 2–3 hours with a warm drink.

Honeysuckle and forsythia are the main ingredients of this formula. They are used to clear mild chills and fever, headache, thirst, and cough. Take as an infusion with 1 tsp of each herb in a pot of boiled water. Sweeten with honey.

SORE THROAT

Often a sore throat is the first indication of a cold. Plenty of rest and drinking lots of liquids should help it to pass quickly. If it continues, and is very painful with swollen glands, there is the chance that it has turned into a throat infection and may need professional treatment.

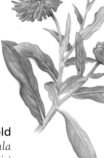

Marigold
(Calendula officinalis)

ECHINACEA, CLEAVERS, AND MARIGOLD

These herbs will help with more persistent and infected sore throats. Echinacea is excellent for fighting infections and is often taken as a tincture. It is advisable for adults to take at least 1 tsp two or three times a day with a severe infection, and it is safe to use in smaller doses for children.

Cleavers and marigold will also help to clear infections from the lymphatic system and can be taken in combination as a tea or tincture.

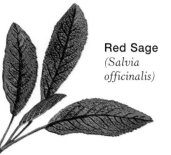

Red Sage
(Salvia officinalis)

RED SAGE

Use this as a gargle by making an infusion of 1 heaping teaspoon of sage in 1 cup of water. You can also drink this as a soothing tea.

COUGHS

There are many different types of coughs, and each type needs its own remedy. Often one type of cough will turn into another one, and this can be very confusing. It is worthwhile trying to find the right remedy because herbs are very good at clearing coughs, especially those that are very persistent. Chronic coughs can indicate a lung weakness which acupuncture may be able to strengthen.

COLTSFOOT, HYSSOP, AND ELECAMPANE

These herbs will help clear a loose, phlegmy cough. Add some echinacea tincture if the catarrh is green; this indicates there is an infection.

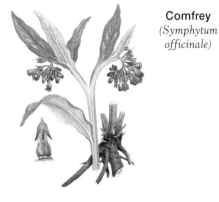

Comfrey
(Symphytum officinale)

GINGER, HONEY, AND LEMON

This traditional remedy is simple but effective in treating coughs with lots of clear mucus.

> ### GOLDEN SEAL
> Is another great herb for moving and drying phlegm. It should be used in smaller doses and *avoided during pregnancy*.

MARSHMALLOW, COLTSFOOT, MULLEIN, AND COMFREY

These herbs will soothe dry, irritating coughs. Add honey or licorice to sweeten and moisten.

THYME AND WILD CHERRY

These herbs are very soothing and useful with spasms of coughing, especially those that keep you awake at night. Thyme can be added to the bath, or use a few drops of thyme oil on your pillow to help relax the lungs.

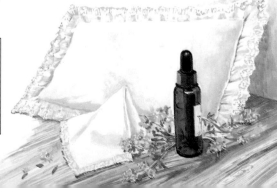

EARACHES

For the initial stages of earache where pain is mild and fever is low or non-existent, the following herbs are very useful. If pain is extreme with a high fever and purulent discharge coming from the ear, it is best to seek medical help immediately. Avoid putting any drops into the ear if the eardrum has burst.

Chamomile
(*Anthemis nobilis*)

Echinacea
(*Echinacea angustifolia*)

CHAMOMILE, SKULLCAP, HYSSOP, AND ECHINACEA

Drink as a medicinal tea three times a day to help clear the infection and soothe the pain.

GARLIC, LAVENDER, AND OLIVE OIL

This mixture makes excellent eardrops. Slice the garlic and place in a small amount of olive oil with a few lavender flowers. Leave for 2 hours. Strain. Warm 1 tsp of the oil by placing it over a cup of hot water. Put a few drops into the sore ear and plug with cotton.

EYE COMPLAINTS

Here are a few suggestions for herbal teas that will help with dry, red, and irritated eyes. If you make an eye wash, it is important to make it as a decoction and to use sterilized containers to prevent infection from spreading.

EYEBRIGHT

This is an excellent herb used to strengthen and heal almost all eye ailments. It can be made into an eye wash or taken internally as a tea. Add chamomile or marigold to help soothe sore eyes. Or use cold chamomile tea bags on the eyes as a simple compress to clear red, irritated eyes.

Eyebright
(*Euphrasia officinalis*)

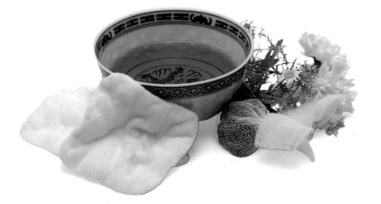

CHRYSANTHEMUM

(*Ju Hua*, Chinese Chrysanthemum)
This is useful for sore, red, irritated eyes. Drink as a tea, use as an eye wash, or make a compress with the tea bags. is also helpful for eye problems related to headaches. Ther is a patent formula called *Qi Ju Di Huang Wan* which contains *Ju Hua*. This helps to strengthen and brighten ey especially if there are feelings of general tiredness. Older people with chronic eye conditions may also find it helpfu

HEADACHES AND MIGRAINE

There are many different types of headaches, with migraines possibly being the most extreme. The cause of the headache is important to sort out. This could be eye strain, back problems, allergies, sinusitis, or hormonal imbalances, to name a few. Tension and overwork can also cause headaches, and if this is the case, try to take some time off for rest and relaxation.

Herbal baths using a strong infusion of oils can make the whole process of unwinding deliciously pleasant! Massaging relaxing oils such as lavender, peppermint, or marjoram into the head, neck, and feet can ease muscle tensions and bring great relief.

Chamomile, feverfew, lavender, lemon balm, marjoram, meadowsweet, peppermint, rosemary, skullcap, thyme, valerian, and vervain are just a few herbs useful for headache pain, depending on the underlying cause. Try them on their own or mix several together. Look them up in the herbal section (pages 8–17) to find out what suits you best.

Herbal baths using a strong infusion of oils can make the whole process of unwinding deliciously pleasant!

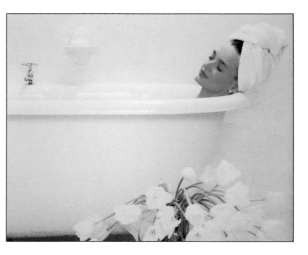

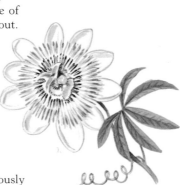

Passion-flower
(Passiflora incarnata)

SKULLCAP, VALERIAN, AND PASSION-FLOWER
Use these very effective herbs for pain relief and to ease stress and tension.

AGNUS CASTUS AND WILD YAM
If headaches are related to the menstrual cycle, these herbs can be added to any listed here. They will need to be taken over several months to re-establish hormonal balance.

Feverfew
(Tanacetum parthenium)

LEMON BALM, LAVENDER, AND MEADOWSWEET
This is a good herbal mixture if the headaches are related to digestive upsets.

Lavender
(Lavandula officinalis)

LEMON BALM, FEVERFEW, MEADOWSWEET, AND ROSEMARY
Combine these herbs in infusions and drink 3 cups daily if you are prone to migraines. Migraines can also be brought on by allergies to certain foods, low blood sugar, stress, hormonal imbalances, and postural problems, so it is important to check these out!

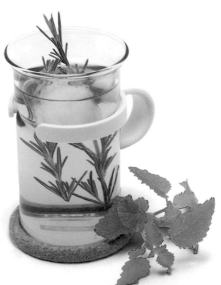

HAY FEVER

Allergies to grasses and pollens can cause great discomfort. To prevent the hay fever from occurring and to be really effective, start treatment a month before your particular hay-fever season begins. This will help to tone up your system before the allergens hit the air, and your nose! It may be necessary to go on a low-mucus diet, avoiding foods which increase catarrh such as cheese, eggs, milk, bananas, and peanut butter. Vitamin C, zinc, and garlic will build up your resistance, so it may help to take these supplements. Acupuncture treatment is also helpful in strengthening and clearing your system so allergic reactions are less severe.

Garlic
(Allium sativum)

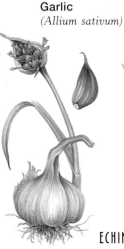

Echinacea
(Echinacea angustifolia)

ECHINACEA, ELDERFLOWER, EYEBRIGHT, AND HYSSOP

Combine in equal quantities and make a tea to drink three times a day.

CHAMOMILE AND EYEBRIGHT

Make a decoction and use it to bathe the eyes.

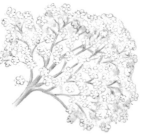

Elderflower
(Sambucus nigra)

Herbal remedies can help to alleviate many of the uncomfortable symptoms which plague allergy sufferers.

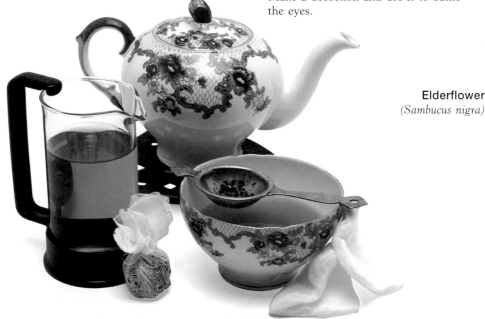

Bi Yan Pian
This Chinese patent remedy is excellent for clearing the congestion of hay fever. Take it with the first symptoms of hay fever and it will help to stop them from developing. It is best to take the pills after meals.

SINUSITIS

Inflammation of the sinus cavities can lead to an overproduction of mucus. This can create pain above or behind the eyes, and stuffiness. Chronic sinusitis can be aggravated by colds, hay fever, and damp weather. A low-mucus diet and supplements (see suggestions for hay fever opposite) is recommended. Acupuncture treatment is also very successful with treating sinusitis. A high fever and severe pain may indicate that there is an infection, and medical help is advised.

ECHINACEA, EYEBRIGHT, ELDERFLOWER, GOLDEN SEAL, AND MARSH MALLOW

These herbs taken as a tea or tincture are very effective at clearing catarrh and soothing irritated membranes in the nose.

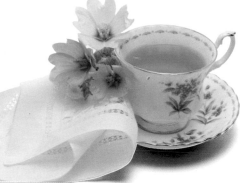

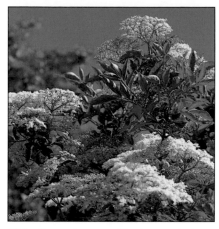

Elderflower is very effective at drying up mucus and fighting infections.

PALPITATIONS

Irregular or forcible heartbeats can have many different causes such as allergies, menopause, fear, sexual excitement, and overconsumption of coffee and cigarettes. Although they can't help the underlying cause (only some behavior changes can do that), herbal remedies can help to reduce erratic and fast heartbeats and stop them from damaging the heart.

LEMON BALM, LIME BLOSSOM, MOTHERWORT, AND PASSION-FLOWER

Take this infusion to help with palpitations with signs of stress and anxiety.

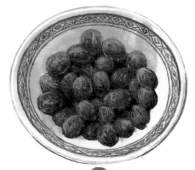

Lime blossom
(Tilia europea)

Motherwort
(Leonurus cardiaca)

HAWTHORN BERRIES

These berries are very helpful in regulating the heartbeat, normalizing heart function, and strengthening the cardiovascular system. Add them if there are any signs of high blood pressure or heart problems.

DIGESTIVE SYSTEM

Eating should be one of life's many pleasures. Problems with digestion can create discomfort which then begins to affect all aspects of daily life. It is best to listen to the body and deal with digestive complaints while symptoms are still mild. This can help to prevent more serious digestive ailments which are often painful, difficult to cure, and very debilitating. Herbs for the more chronic condition of irritable bowel syndrome are suggested, although this may need professional treatment.

A healthy diet and regular meals are important means of helping any problem that relates to digestion, and this is an essential part of treatment. Good digestion thrives on relaxed, peaceful mealtimes. In addition to eating healthily and regularly, take some time to enjoy your food.

INDIGESTION AND HEARTBURN

Stomach discomfort, gas, and acidity can be the result of too many rich, fatty, or spicy foods; drinking too much tea, coffee, or alcohol; or smoking cigarettes. Stress, tension, and rushed meals can also affect the digestion. If you already eat in a healthy, regular, and relaxed manner and still feel unwell, try the following herbal remedies.

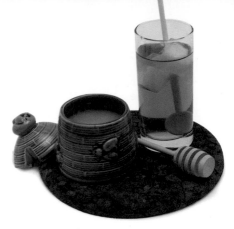

Meadowsweet
(Filipendula ulmaria)

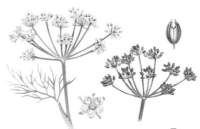

Fennel
(Foeniculum vulgare)

CARDAMOM, PEPPERMINT, AND FENNEL
Take these herbs after eating to aid digestion and settle the stomach. They also help to clear gas and bloating. The traditional after-dinner mint or Indian cardamom tea may be based on this knowledge.

SLIPPERY ELM
This can be taken in tablet form or powder and has the effect of soothing the stomach lining. Take the powder mixed in hot water and sweetened with honey. It has an unusual taste and texture, but does work very well to ease acid indigestion and stop pain. It is also very nourishing to the digestive system.

MEADOWSWEET, COMFREY, AND MARSH MALLOW
These herbs also help to heal a sensitive stomach lining. Take as a combination or individually.

CHAMOMILE, ROSEMARY, AND LEMON BALM
These relaxing herbs aid digestion and are especially useful if there is susceptibility to nervous upsets.

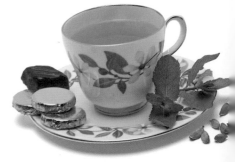

NAUSEA

Nausea can be the result of many different conditions, and once again, it is important to establish the underlying cause.

GINGER, CHAMOMILE, FENNEL, AND PEPPERMINT

To help settle the stomach, try sipping these herbal teas slowly. They are all mild, safe herbs so they can be used with children for travel sickness and illness. They are also fine to use for morning sickness for pregnant women. Try peppermints or ginger snaps for a treat.

TANGERINE PEEL (*Chen Pi*)

This fragrant Chinese herb has many uses for digestive disorders and eases nausea as well as feelings of fullness and bloating. It helps to strengthen the digestion and send the food downward. Take as a tea or a tincture in warm water after meals. It is interesting that citrus peel is used in the West in rich fruit cakes, maybe to help us digest them better!

LEMON BALM, HOPS, AND PASSION-FLOWER

These herbs will help to calm the stomach and are useful if nervous tension is present. Usually they are taken with some of the herbs listed here as either a tea or a tincture.

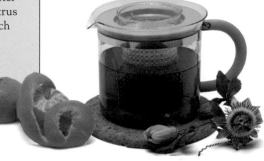

ABDOMINAL PAIN AND BLOATING

Abdominal pain and bloating can be indications of a variety of digestive disturbances. It is important to understand the underlying cause which can be anything from a weak, nervous digestion, food allergies, or bad eating habits, to more complicated conditions such as ulcers, gallstones, or irritable bowel syndrome.

If a person has food sensitivities, certain herbs may be aggravating. Use them in small amounts at first. Daily massage of the lower abdomen, in a clockwise direction starting from the center and moving outward may help. There is also a wide variety of nutritional supplements that aid digestion.

WILD YAM, PEPPERMINT, GINGER, CINNAMON, FENNEL, LEMON BALM, AND CHAMOMILE

These herbs are good for clearing gas and easing bloating. Drink a cup of one of these herbal teas after meals, or take a few drops of the tincture in some warm water.

Cayenne

Caraway seeds

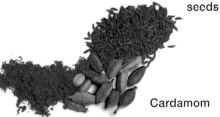

Cardamom

CAYENNE, GINGER, CARDAMOM, AND CARAWAY SEEDS

Add these warming spices to your cooking, but avoid using them if you are suffering from ulcers or irritable bowel syndrome.

Ginger
(*Zingiber offinale*)

Xiang Sha Liu Jun Wan
This Chinese patent formula contains herbs to strengthen the digestion and alleviate pain and distension. It is also indicated for reduced appetite, feelings of fullness after eating small amounts, belching, and sometimes nausea and diarrhea. Avoid using long term if there is thirst, irritability, and constipation as it may be too warming.

CONSTIPATION

Constipation is not a disease, but a symptom of other problems. A good diet should include foods that contain fiber. This is found in many fruits and vegetables as well as in whole-wheat bread, cereals, nuts, and seeds. Avoid refined foods such as white bread, cakes, and candy. Dairy products, especially hard cheeses, can also be clogging. Stress and tension affect the digestion, and there may be a tendency to "hold on" to things psychologically and physically Relaxation classes or a break from your usual routines may be a positive solution.

Medication may have constipation as a side effect, and it is always important to be aware of this when taking any drugs. Long-term use of laxatives is potentially harmful to the digestion as they do not encourage the peristaltic movement of the intestines and may "push" the food through without its goodness being absorbed fully. As with most digestive problems, it is important to eat regularly and drink plenty of liquids. Physical exercise, even walking, will help to keep the system moving.

WATER AND LEMON JUICE

This simple combination taken first thing in the morning, half an hour before any food is eaten, can really help and is worth trying!

PSYLLIUM SEEDS AND LINSEED

Put 1–2 tsp of seeds in a cup of hot water. Let them soak for 2 hours. Sweeten with lemon and honey and drink. Alternatively, sprinkle the seeds on cereal for breakfast. Linseeds are also rich in oils that are used to help moisturize hair and skin, so they have the added benefit of enhancing beauty!

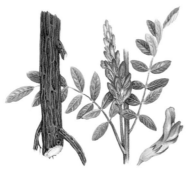

Licorice
(Glycyrrhiza glabra)

RHUBARB ROOT

Taken in small doses, it helps to tone the intestines and promote appetite. In large doses, it purges – this should be avoided except in extreme cases. Please note that this is not the same as garden rhubarb, and that it may color the urine yellow or red. *Use with caution in pregnancy, definitely avoiding large doses.*

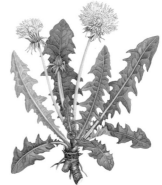

Dandelion root
(Taraxacum officinale)

LICORICE, GINGER, DANDELION ROOT, YELLOW DOCK ROOT, AND BURDOCK

If constipation does not respond to changes in diet and the suggestions above, try a mixture of these herbs. Substitute fennel for ginger if there is a lot of gas and colic.

DIARRHEA

This condition may be due to an acute gastric infection, or it may be more long term in cases where there is a weakness in the digestive system. Stress, anxiety, and new situations may also affect the bowels, causing diarrhea. Generally, it is best to eat plain foods and avoid alcohol, coffee, dairy products, and spicy or rich foods. Better still, in acute cases, try to avoid eating for 24 hours, but drink plenty of liquids and teas. If the diarrhea is severe or persistent, it is necessary to get medical help, especially with children. With bouts of diarrhea, it may be necessary to re-mineralize the body and taking "Dioralyte" will help replace lost mineral salts and prevent dehydration. Water, mixed with small amounts of baking soda and sugar, will also work.

MEADOWSWEET

Take frequently as a tea or tincture. It will help to settle the stomach and stop diarrhea. It is safe to use with children.

CHAMOMILE AND LEMON BALM

These herbs are used to help relaxation and can be added to meadowsweet to ease diarrhea due to anxiety and nervousness.

> *Si Jun Zi Tang*
> ("Four gentlemen decoction")
> This Chinese prescription can be taken as a decoction, tincture, or powder. It is mild in nature and is strengthening to the digestion and general energy. It is best taken over a long period of time.

BAYBERRY, AGRIMONY, AND COMFREY ROOT

This mixture is useful to stop diarrhea in adults. Add root ginger and camomile to soothe griping pains. Add marsh mallow to help ease symptoms of acidity and inflammation.

SAGE

Drink sage tea after a light meal to aid digestion and reduce diarrhea.

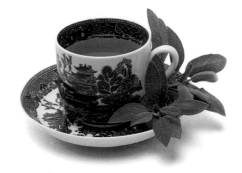

IRRITABLE BOWEL SYNDROME

This common complaint has varying symptoms for each individual who suffers from it. Often there is alternating diarrhea and constipation with flatulence and discomfort. It may be a result of stress and bad eating habits. It could also be caused by allergic reactions to certain foods. These food intolerances are different with each person, but common ones are tea, coffee, wheat, and dairy products. It is often difficult to discover food allergies, and even more difficult to avoid them, especially if they are ones found in commonly eaten foods such as wheat.

The best procedure is to cut out one food at a time for 10 days. Gradually reintroduce it back into the diet, noting any reactions. It may be best to consult a nutritionist, especially if allergies are severe.

SLIPPERY ELM

This is a favorite for most digestive problems because it is soothing and nourishing. Take three times a day as a gruel using 1 tsp per cup of hot water. Sweeten with honey.

WILD YAM, CHAMOMILE, PEPPERMINT, AGRIMONY, MARSH MALLOW, AND GOLDEN SEAL

Drink a cup of these herbs three to six times a day to soothe the bowel and stop inflammation. Add the golden seal as a tincture as the smell of the powder can make it unpleasant to drink. *Do not use golden seal if you are pregnant as it stimulates the uterus.*

LIME BLOSSOM, SKULLCAP, AND HOPS

Add one or more of these herbs to the above mixture for Irritable Bowel Syndrome if stress is increasing bowel problems. Avoid using hops if suffering from depression.

REPRODUCTIVE AND URINARY SYSTEMS

Most women's lives will be affected by changes in their reproductive systems. The onset of menstruation, pregnancy and birth, and the time of the menopause are strong influences over their feelings of sexuality and growth. They may be the markers of important cycles of change.

In this section herbs are included that will help women to adjust to these changes more easily. In addition, there are some useful herbs for cystitis, which is not necessarily linked to the reproductive system, but is common in women.

PREMENSTRUAL SYNDROME

Premenstrual syndrome (PMS) is widely recognized today, and it is generally accepted that hormones can affect emotional states. The symptoms and duration of PMS will vary from woman to woman. Symptoms can include emotional instability, lack of coordination, water retention, painful breasts, headaches, nausea, and skin changes (see relevant sections on pages 33 and 46).

Diet supplements, like evening primrose oil, magnesium, calcium, and vitamin B, may be useful. Acupuncture treatment taken over several months is very effective and a great way to unwind.

AGNUS CASTUS

This herb helps to stabilize the hormones. Combine and make a decoction to drink three times a day as a course of treatment for three months. Tinctures and pills are also available and easier to use. It is important to take this herb daily.

MOTHERWORT, SKULLCAP, AND PASSION-FLOWER

These herbs help to ease feelings of stress and anxiety. Decoct valerian root, or add as a tincture, if there is muscle tension through the neck and shoulders, but avoid long-term use of this herb.

Xiao Yao San
This Chinese patent formula helps to ease general symptoms of PMS, especially if there are digestive problems the week before the period. If there are symptoms of weakness and tiredness, take "Women's precious pills" (see page 17) when the bleeding has stopped. Continue these until the week before the period, when *Xiao Yao San* is taken again. Take the combination of patent formulas for three months to help regulate the menstrual cycle.

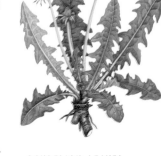

Dandelion
(Taraxacum officinale)

Parsley
(Petroselinum crispum)

DANDELION LEAVES AND PARSLEY

These herbs will act as a diuretic to ease water retention. Combine and infuse to make a tea to be drunk when needed.

DYSMENORRHEA

Painful periods are a very common complaint. Most often, the pain is disruptive and uncomfortable, and herbs can be a natural way of easing it. Pain at the beginning of the bleeding is often due to the reduction of blood flow by spasms of the uterus. Pain lasting throughout the period is more often due to congestion within the uterus. If pain is severely uncomfortable, if there is heavy bleeding, or if there are signs of infection mid-cycle (i.e., if there is pain, fever, or smelly discharge), it is important to seek medical advice immediately and consult a qualified herbal practitioner.

AGNUS CASTUS, FALSE UNICORN ROOT, MOTHERWORT, AND SQUAW VINE

These herbs help to balance the hormones and to tonify the uterus. Combine and drink three times a day for six weeks.

Marigold
(*Calendula officinalis*)

WILD YAM, CRAMPBARK, PASQUE FLOWER, MARIGOLD, AND RASPBERRY LEAF

For period pain, combine and drink three times a day when needed.

RASPBERRY LEAF, MARIGOLD, NETTLE, AND SHEPHERD'S PURSE

For heavy bleeding or bleeding between periods, pour a cup of boiling water on to 1–2 tsp of dried herbs. Infuse for 10 minutes and drink every 2–3 hours just before and during a period.

GINGER, CINNAMON, AND CLOVES

Pain can also be due to cold, and these pungent herbs can warm the uterus and help the blood to flow more easily. Add them to a tea, or better still, make a mulled wine.

AMENORRHEA

Amenorrhea is the condition in which menstruation does not occur. This can be due to physical exhaustion, stress and anxiety, weight loss for any reason, hormonal dysfunction, or when stopping use of the contraceptive pill (because the body may take some time to regain its natural rhythms). However, it may also be due to an underlying physical condition. Because of this, and because these herbs might harm an unknown pregnancy, *it is extremely important that you check with your doctor before using any of these remedies, to be sure that you are healthy and not pregnant.*

PENNYROYAL AND TANSY

For treating regular menstrual cycle with occasionally delayed menstruation, infuse and drink three times a day until the period begins.

AGNUS CASTUS, FALSE UNICORN ROOT, BLUE COHOSH, RUE, AND MOTHERWORT

These herbs will help to regulate hormonal activity, strengthen the uterus, and bring on delayed or suppressed menstruation. Decoct and drink three times a day.

DANG GUI BU XUE TANG

This Chinese patent remedy helps to nourish the blood. Take over several months if there is anemia, paleness, and tiredness with little or no menstrual bleeding.

Pennyroyal
(*Mentha pulegium*)

LICORICE, BLACK COHOSH, AGNUS CASTUS, AND MOTHERWORT

If stopping use of the contraceptive pill, these herbs will benefit the adrenal glands, tone the uterus, and normalize hormonal function. After coming off the pill, decoct and drink three times a day for the first week, twice a day for the second week, and once a day for the third week.

Rue
(*Ruta graveolens*)

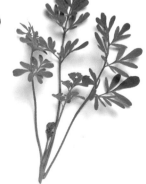

INFERTILITY

Problems in conceiving are on the increase, and it is well worth trying acupuncture, homeopathy, and herbal and nutritional therapies. A qualified practitioner should be consulted if you do not have good results with these herbs after several months.

DAMIANA, SAW PALMETTO, CELERY SEEDS, OATS, LICORICE, AND GINGER

These herbs will help to raise a low sperm count and help to strengthen the male reproductive system. It is also important to eat well, and avoid alcohol, cigarettes, caffeine, tight clothes, and hot baths.

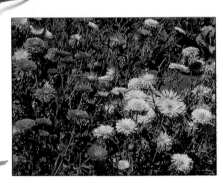

FALSE UNICORN ROOT, ROSES, NETTLE, AND MARIGOLD

These herbs will help to balance hormones and nourish the blood and uterus. Take over several months and follow the advice suggested above. Vitamin B, royal jelly, Floradix, kelp, and evening primrose oil may also be helpful, depending on your state of health.

Rose
(Rosa gallica)

Nettle
(Urtica dioica)

Marigold
(Calendula officinalis)

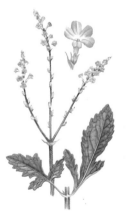

Vervain
(Verbena officinalis)

NETTLE, SKULLCAP, VERVAIN, DANDELION ROOT, AND PRICKLY ASH

For low vitality and stress, add a combination of these herbs to enhance the effects of those listed above.

PREGNANCY, BIRTH, AND POSTNATAL CARE

Herbal treatment for pregnancy, birth, and postnatal care has a very rich and valuable tradition. For centuries, midwives have used herbs to help women maintain a healthy pregnancy, ease birth, and support postnatal care. Many of the herbs used in this section for the healing of women and aiding the birthing process have come from the different tribes of the Native Americans. Herbs such as squaw vine, black cohosh, blue cohosh, and false unicorn root are invaluable complements to European remedies. While it is best to avoid medication with pregnancy, some herbs may be very beneficial.

HERBS TO BE AVOIDED DURING PREGNANCY:

Some herbs have a stimulating action on the uterus which may result in miscarriage, the most common of which are aloes, autumn crocus, barberry, golden seal, juniper, male fern, mandrake, pennyroyal, poke root, rhubarb, rue, sage, southernwood, tansy, thuja, and wormwood.

CHAMOMILE, LEMON BALM, AND MEADOWSWEET

A mixture of these herbs, or the use of any one of them, may help to settle the stomach if suffering from morning sickness. Take as an infusion when needed.

PEPPERMINT, FENNEL, GINGER, AND CINNAMON

These herbs are warming to the digestion and may also help to settle the stomach if suffering from morning sickness. Take the peppermint or fennel alone, or add any one of these herbs to another tea. For example, try adding a couple of slices of root ginger to a pot of meadowsweet tea.

RASPBERRY LEAF AND SQUAW VINE

These herbs help to strengthen the uterus and prepare for birth. Take 1 tsp of one herb or combine ½ tsp of both herbs per cup and drink an infusion once or twice a day during the last three months of pregnancy.

BLACK COHOSH, BLUE COHOSH, AND GOLDEN SEAL

These herbs help to strengthen weak contractions during labor. Take a mixture with some ginger.

BLUE COHOSH, WILD YAM, CRAMPBARK, RASPBERRY LEAVES, AND SQUAW VINE

For short, sharp contractions during labor with tension and pain and a rigid cervix, take these herbs as a tea or tincture.

Nu Ke Ba Zhen Wan ("Women's precious pills") Take 5 tablets three times a day to help revitalize and nourish after the birth.

COMFREY, MARIGOLD, AND ST. JOHN'S WORT

Use 1 tbsp of herbs to 1 pint (500ml) of water for a soothing and healing bath after the birth.

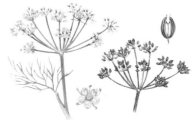

Fennel
(Foeniculum vulgare)

NETTLES, FENNEL, VERVAIN, BORAGE, RASPBERRY LEAVES, OR MARSH MALLOW

Take any of these herbs individually or in combination to help increase milk production. Drink one cup three times a day.

CHINESE ANGELICA AND ASTRAGALUS

These two herbs in combination help to nourish the blood and strengthen the *Qi* (vital force). This is especially important if the labor has been long and difficult, or there has been much loss of blood. Traditionally, the *Dang Gui* was cooked with a chicken, and the meat and juices were used to nourish the new mother. The herbs also come prepared as a patent formula called *Dang Gui Bu Xue Tang*.

COMFREY, CHICKWEED, OR MARIGOLD-CALENDULA OINTMENTS

Rub into sore, cracked nipples for relief.

MENOPAUSAL DISCOMFORTS

Menopause is an important time of change and transition. Its onset may be gradual, with periods coming less frequently, or it may occur quite suddenly. In most cases, there are also many emotional adjustments to make. Issues such as aging, children leaving home, and career decisions may need to be faced. Physically, there are changes in the pituitary and ovarian hormone levels due to the ovaries no longer releasing the ovum. Discomforts commonly experienced are hot flashes, palpitations, irritability, depression, insomnia, joint pain, and general debility. Any severe discomforts or excessive bleeding require medical attention. Constitutional treatment and emotional support from a qualified practitioner or therapist may be useful.

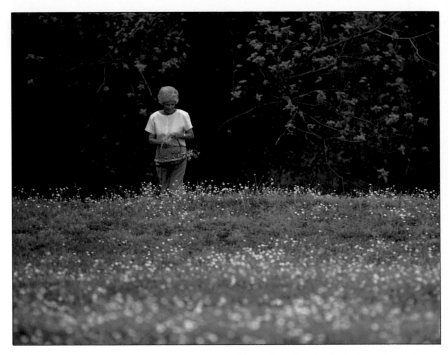

SAGE AND BLACKCURRANT LEAVES

These herbs taken as a tea will help to reduce symptoms of hot flashes.

AGNUS CASTUS, FALSE UNICORN ROOT, WILD YAM, ST. JOHN'S WORT, CHINESE ANGELICA, AND MOTHERWORT

Herbal combination used to establish a new level of hormonal function.
Decoct and drink three times a day for three months.

By easing the physical discomforts that may occur during menopause, an older woman can cope with other changes in her life.

Sage
(Salvia officinalis)

SKULLCAP, VERVAIN, AND LIME BLOSSOM

Use this gentle herbal combination to ease nervousness, anxiety, depression, and mood swings. They may be added to other herbal combinations, depending on your symptoms.

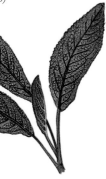

Chinese angelica
(Radix angelicae sinensis)

Cystitis

This urinary tract infection can be caused by inflammation in the bladder and/or urethra. Symptoms may be an urgency and frequency of urination, with pain or a burning sensation. Drink plenty of water, adding 1 tsp of baking soda twice a day. *Do not do this if you have a heart problem.*
Avoid coffee, tea, alcohol, spicy foods, citrus fruits, and cigarettes. If there is fever, low back pain, bloody or cloudy urine, it is important to get medical attention as there is a chance of a kidney infection. If you have recurrent bouts of cystitis, professional help may be needed.

BARLEY WATER

Simmer 4 oz. (113g) of washed pot barley in 1 pint (500ml) of water until the barley is soft. Strain and add honey and lemon. Drink as needed.

BUCHU, CORNSILK, COUCHGRASS, AND MARSH MALLOW LEAVES

Combine, infuse, and drink a cupful every two hours.

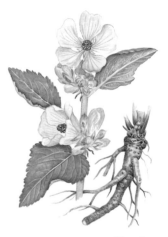

Marsh mallow
(Althaea officinalis)

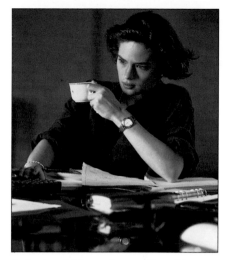

Irritating drinks such as coffee will increase the pain and inflammation in the bladder.

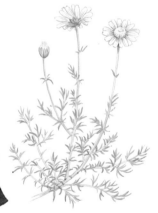

Chamomile
(Anthemis nobilis)

WHOLE BODY AND SKIN

This section covers ailments which may affect the whole body. To treat these conditions effectively, the body has to be led back to a state of health and balance. One of the major causes of rheumatism and arthritis is the accumulation of toxins or waste products in the joints. Although only one or two joints may be painful, it may be necessary to look at what is going on in the whole body in order to find a cure.

Fatigue, tiredness, and aching muscles can also be due to the body, gradually becoming more toxic and sensitive to foods, pollution, and stress. Myalgic encephalomyelitis (ME), post-viral syndrome, and chronic Epstein Barr virus disease are all conditions in which fatigue is the major disability. Their causes are not clear, but complementary medicine can offer relief and hope.

ARTHRITIS AND RHEUMATISM

These painful conditions have many forms varying from hot, swollen, painful joints to stiff and difficult movements. It may be necessary to have a good osteopathic treatment to check the alignment of the bones and muscles.

Food allergies can eventually cause a buildup of toxicity in the joints. Acidic reactions are caused by red meat, eggs, dairy products, vinegar, pickles, refined sugars, and most spices. Foods rich in oxalic acid, such as rhubarb, gooseberries, and red currants, should also be avoided. Coffee, black tea, alcohol, sugar, and salt can also contribute to the accumulation of toxins, and are detrimental to a cleansing process. Instead eat plenty of whole grains and vegetables (exclude tomatoes, although this is technically a fruit). Drink at least 3 pints (1.8l) of water/liquid a day to flush the system. Take cod liver oil, evening primrose oil, kelp, and selenium to help repair bones and cartilage.

Finally, it is worth mentioning that our body is affected by our mental state. Stress and tension can restrict our movements and circulation, stopping muscles and joints from getting the exercise and blood flow that they need. Yoga, Tai Chi, and any other gentle activity will help increase mobility and alleviate stiffness. Acupuncture can also be very effective in removing pain and stiffness. As with any other ailment, if you are in a great deal of pain and discomfort, please seek professional medical care.

CELERY SEED, BURDOCK, MEADOWSWEET, AND YARROW

These herbs help to cleanse the system. Take this tea over a long period of time.

BLACK COHOSH AND BLUE COHOSH

Add to the tea if symptoms are post-menopausal to help balance the hormones.

YELLOW DOCK AND LICORICE

Constipation can increase the build-up of toxicity, making regular bowel movements important. If this is a problem, add these herbs to the celery seed, burdock, meadowsweet, and yarrow tea.

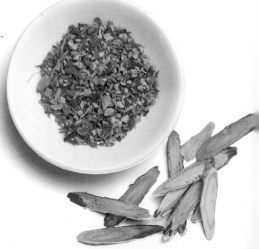

Yellow dock root
and Licorice

JAMAICAN DOGWOOD, PASSION-FLOWER, AND VALERIAN

These herbs will help if pain is preventing sleep. Take this tea or tincture half an hour before bedtime. It is a safe mixture and may be used in a slightly stronger dose than normal. *Avoid long-term use of valerian.*

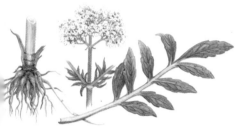

Valerian
(Valeriana officinalis)

NETTLE, HAWTHORN, AND PRICKLY ASH

These herbs help improve circulation. Add to other herbs or use on their own if pain and stiffness have gone.

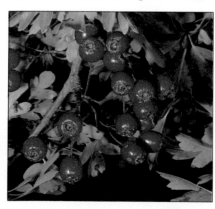

Hawthorn *(Crataegus oxyacanthoides)*

Passion-flower
(Passiflora incarnata)

Peppermint
(Mentha piperata)

ST. JOHN'S WORT, PEPPERMINT, AND LAVENDER OILS

Massage painful joints with these oils to help increase circulation and ease pain.

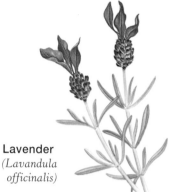

Lavender
(Lavandula officinalis)

GREEN CABBAGE LEAVES AND COMFREY LEAVES

Wrap hot, swollen, painful joints in these to help relieve swelling and pain.

CHRONIC TIREDNESS AND FATIGUE

Chronic tiredness can be the result of many different conditions. In order to treat it effectively, it is important to find out the cause, or at least eliminate some of the possibilities! A physical examination by a doctor, including blood tests, is necessary especially if the fatigue is severe. Take a good look at the possibility of overworking and emotional stress being the causes. Maybe it is important to take a long-overdue holiday. Depression and fatigue are sometimes linked, and it is hard to tell which came first. Try to sort out any long-term stressful situations (see section on Emotions, pages 52–5). If tiredness is coming in waves during the day, it may be due to low blood sugar or food allergies.

Eating healthy, regular meals and avoiding excesses of caffeine, alcohol, and sugar may be difficult to do at first, but well worth it in the long run. Sleeping difficulties need to be addressed so that you wake rested and refreshed (see Insomnia, page 54). Regular exercise can help you to keep fit and strong. For many people, especially those with sedentary jobs, exercise has been found very revitalizing. However, if exercise makes you feel even more exhausted, stop doing it. ME, post-viral syndrome, and chronic Epstein-Barr virus have symptoms which will vary with each individual, but are generally made worse from exercise and lack of rest. Their acute phase may be like flu, which then develops into a more debilitating condition, the symptoms including fatigue, muscular aches, poor memory and concentration, sore throats, dizziness, and digestive complaints.

Finally, if you are on any medication, check for any side effects of tiredness. The dosage or the drug may need to be altered, but always check with the doctor first.

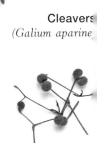

Cleavers
(Galium aparine)

Echinacea
(Echinacea angustifolia)

ECHINACEA, YELLOW DOCK ROOT, CLEAVERS, MARIGOLD, AND LICORICE

These herbs will help to cleanse the body and enhance the immune system. They are appropriate to take when tiredness is due to poor diet, over-indulgences in alcohol and caffeine, smoking, recurring infections, ME, or candidiasis. They can be taken as tea or tincture three times a day over several months if necessary.

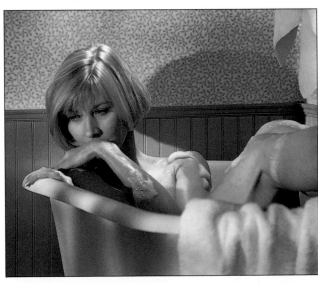

Putting soothing herbs in the bath can aid restful sleep.

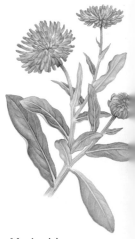

Marigold
(Calendula officinalis)

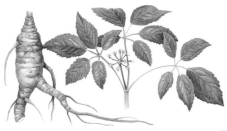

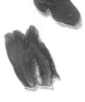

Ginseng
(Radix ginseng)

GINSENG

This Chinese herb is renowned for its strengthening properties. It is very useful with any debility and can be taken for three-month periods. *Avoid if pregnant or with high blood pressure.* Use only if there is debility; it is inappropriate to use if you are well.

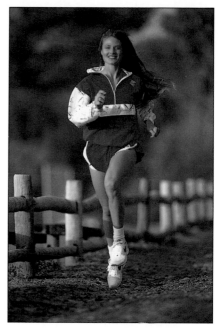

Regular exercise can be revitalizing by helping to release stress and tension and increase the blood flow to all parts of the body.

Si Jun Zi Tang
("Four gentlemen decoction")
This Chinese herbal formula is helpful to rebuild strength after a debilitating illness. Take as a decoction over a long period of time.

OATS, VERVAIN, AND DANDELION

These herbs support the nervous system and help to cleanse the liver. They would be useful as a support after periods of stress and overwork.

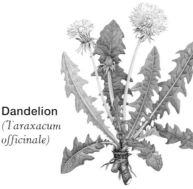

Dandelion
(Taraxacum officinale)

Yu Ping Feng San
("Jade windscreen powder")
This Chinese herbal formula contains the herb astragalus (*Huang Qi*), which is being used to build up the immune system in chronic conditions like AIDS. The formula can be taken as a decoction, powder, or tincture, and is very useful as a protection against colds and flu.

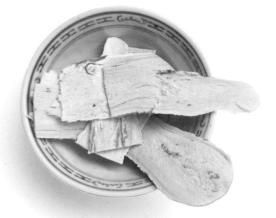

Astragalus
(Radix astragali membranaceus)

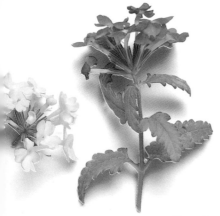

Vervain
(Verbena officinalis)

SKIN CONDITIONS

The skin is a major organ which has the responsibility of protecting you from environmental factors and helps to eliminate internal waste products. Its condition can be affected by sun, age, foods, soaps, and many other things. Here are a few suggestions for the treatment of common skin conditions. Some conditions, such as eczema and psoriasis, may need consultation with a trained herbal practitioner.

ECZEMA

There are many causes of eczema, and these need to be investigated carefully. Allergic reactions to soaps, materials, animals, and foods can aggravate it. Stress can also cause it to flare up. Underlying the condition may be some nutritional deficiencies.
It may be helpful to take evening primrose oil and a multivitamin and mineral supplement.

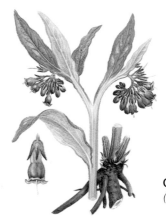

Comfrey
(Symphytum officinale)

RED CLOVER, BORAGE, BURDOCK ROOT, AND NETTLES

This is a basic remedy which can help heal the skin by cleansing and nourishing the blood. It is safe to use with children (see page 19, for correct dosage).

Borage
(Borago officinalis)

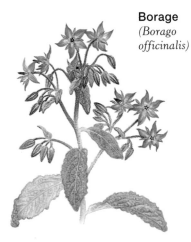

BURDOCK, CHICKWEED, COMFREY, AND MARIGOLD

These herbs can be made into compresses or ointments to soothe irritated skin.

Marigold
(Calendula officinalis)

PSORIASIS

Psoriasis is a common skin complaint which has many different causes, ranging from food allergies to stress and shock. It is important to sort out the underlying causes and treat them accordingly. Often sunshine and sea water will clear psoriasis, although this may be only a temporary solution.

BURDOCK, CLEAVERS, SARSAPARILLA, AND YELLOW DOCK

A decoction of these herbs will help cleanse and strengthen the system if taken over a period of time. Dandelion and red clover can also be used.

SKULLCAP, MOTHERWORT, AND LIME BLOSSOM

Use one or two of these herbs if there are any symptoms of stress, such as palpitations or high blood pressure. Add them to the burdock, cleavers, sarsaparilla, and yellow dock tea.

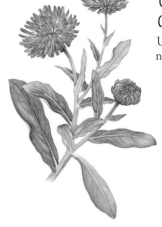

COMFREY AND CHICKWEED OINTMENTS

Use these externally to help nourish and soften the skin.

ACNE

Acne is a common problem for most adolescents, but it can also continue into later years. Often it is hormonally related, which explains its predominance in teenage years and its aggravation before the menstrual cycle. A poor diet of greasy, fried foods or excesses of sugar may also cause an acute attack. These should be avoided and replaced by fresh fruits and vegetables.

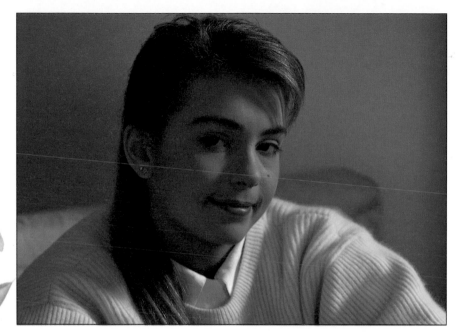

Echinacea
(Echinacea angustifolia)

BURDOCK, CLEAVERS, DANDELION, ECHINACEA, RED CLOVER, AND YELLOW DOCK

These herbs will help to cleanse the system and clear the skin. Drink one cupful three times a day for at least three weeks.

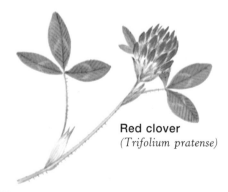

Red clover
(Trifolium pratense)

CHICKWEED, ELDERFLOWER, AND MARIGOLD

Combine in equal parts and use as a facial steam.

Herbal treatment can be very effective in helping adolescents keep a clear, radiant complexion.

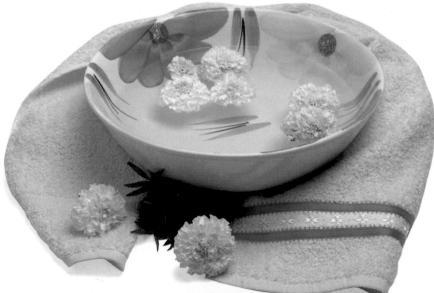

EMOTIONS

In today's society, there is often pressure to get far too much done in too little time. It is not surprising that stress and anxiety levels are so high, often having physical effects such as headaches, indigestion, backache, and many other complaints. Moderate levels of stress and anxiety can turn into chronic depression when people are trapped in situations they feel incapable of changing. People suffering from anxiety, stress, or depression for extended periods of time can become tired and unable to cope with the simple tasks of day-to-day life, and they may eventually experience more serious conditions such as nervous exhaustion or a breakdown. Although herbs cannot eradicate the roots of psychological discomfort, they can temporarily alleviate tension, leaving you more relaxed, steadier and brighter – more capable of creating positive changes.

STRESS AND ANXIETY

Stress and anxiety are responses to a difficult situation. Positively, they can help to bring out the best in a person. If the situation does not change, or continues over a long period, the stress of coping with it can be very debilitating. During periods of stress, your body uses up nutrients faster than usual. Here are some herbs that will help you to feel stronger and calmer. Use them instead of tea and coffee, which contain caffeine.

Lemon Balm
(Melissa officinalis)

VERVAIN, SKULLCAP, OATS, AND GINSENG

These herbs are general tonics for the nervous system. Taken individually or in combination, these herbs will help support a person through a stressful period.

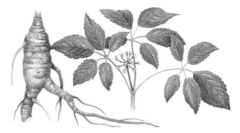

Ginseng
(Radix ginseng)

CHAMOMILE, LIME BLOSSOM, LEMON BALM, AND MEADOWSWEET

Drink these herbs instead of coffee or tea to ease any digestive upsets due to nervous tension.

Meadowsweet
(Filipendula ulmaria)

Hops
(Humulus lupulus)

CHAMOMILE, VALERIAN, HOPS, AND PASSION-FLOWER

These herbs help ease muscle tension and can be mixed with others for stress, anxiety, and depression. Avoid prolonged use of valerian.

DEPRESSION

Depression is another way of reacting to the stresses of life, whether from long-term situations or past causes. Psychotherapy or counseling may help sort out the roots of the problem and provide the individual with the tools to move forward. Exercise, positive self-images, and enjoyable social contacts are also beneficial. If the depression is postnatal or connected with the menstrual cycle, include herbs such as agnus castus and wild yam to help balance the hormones. If it occurs after a long illness, use herbs to build up your body.

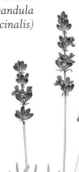

Lavender
(Lavandula officinalis)

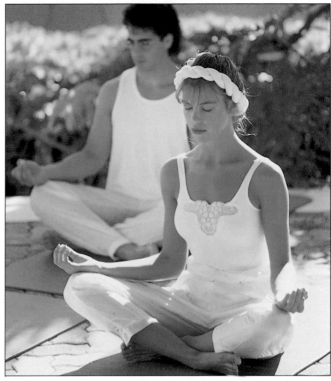

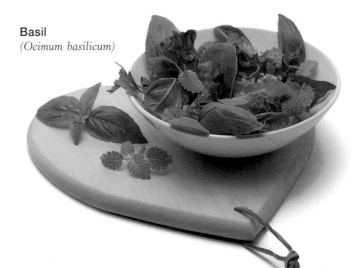

Yoga, positive self-images, and enjoyable social contacts are also beneficial.

GINSENG, LAVENDER, OATS, AND ROSEMARY

If the depression is connected with general debility, this mixture of herbs will be beneficial.

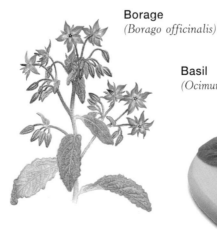

Rosemary
(Rosmarinus officinalis)

Borage
(Borago officinalis)

Basil
(Ocimum basilicum)

LEMON BALM, BORAGE, LIME BLOSSOM, BASIL, ST. JOHN'S WORT, AND SKULLCAP

Any of these herbs can be used alone or in combination to help brighten the mood.

INSOMNIA

Most people will suffer from an occasional night of disturbed sleep. It can happen at a particularly exciting or stressful time. But when it happens often, or when the worry about going to sleep perpetuates insomnia, it becomes problematic. It can be helpful to establish a routine with regular bedtimes and a relaxing before-bed regime. Avoid stimulating activities in the evening, try a peaceful meditation or some gentle exercise, and substitute relaxing herbal teas for caffeine drinks.

Long Yan Rou (Longan fruit) Commonly used in China for insomnia associated with overwork and pensiveness. This is a sweet dried fruit similar to raisins which can be eaten or made into a tea. Take 5–15g a day.

SKULLCAP, VALERIAN, PASSION-FLOWER, AND HOPS

These herbs can be taken as decoctions, tinctures, or pills, and are stronger in their sleep-inducing action, especially in combination with each other. They are useful to break more stubborn patterns of sleeplessness or if pain is causing insomnia.

Avoid prolonged use of valerian, and avoid hops if there are signs of depression.

LEMON BALM, CHAMOMILE, LIME BLOSSOM, AND PASSION-FLOWER

These make excellent nighttime teas to be drunk in the evening before bed. Lime blossom and chamomile can be made into baths for children (see page 23, in Basic Principles).

SKULLCAP, VALERIAN, AND HOPS

These can be made into baths for adults (see page 23, Basic Principles).

Tian Wang Bu Xin Dan ("Emperor of Heaven's special pill to tonify the heart") This Chinese patent remedy is used for insomnia with restless sleep, irritability, fatigue, short concentration, forgetfulness which may be accompanied by mouth ulcers, night sweats, and constipation. It is especially useful for those who have taken sleeping tablets for so long that they have ceased to be effective. Interestingly, the author of this formula reported that it came to him in a dream from the Emperor of Heaven. In Chinese medicine, most sleep disorders are linked with a disturbance in the spirit of the heart, so this is why the heart is mentioned in the English translation of its name.

HYPERACTIVITY

Hyperactivity in children is difficult to define or diagnose. Poor concentration, inability to stay still, and fits of anger or frustration may be symptoms that can be helped by careful diet, patience, and a few herbs. Avoid all foods containing artificial colorings, additives, and sugars. Avoid over-stimulating activities such as computer games and some television programs. Encourage physical activities and lots of fresh air.

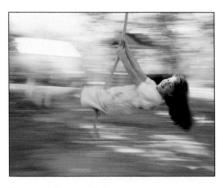

Fun, outdoor activities can help to ease a child's frustrations and use up excess energy.

RED CLOVER

This herb will be safe to use with children over several months and is useful for clearing the body (some people believe hyperactivity is a result of chemical buildup in the body). It also helps to relax the nerves.

OATS AND VITAMINS C AND B-COMPLEX

These will help repair the nervous system which is under strain due to the hyperactivity.

NERVOUS EXHAUSTION

Nervous exhaustion may occur with long-term emotional conflicts, overwork, overconsumption of tea, coffee, and alcohol, and smoking. During stressful periods, vitamins and minerals are used up by the body in higher concentrations. Yet it is often difficult to keep up a healthy diet for various reasons when under stress. You may drink more caffeine and alcohol and smoke more tobacco, all of which cause minerals to be further depleted and put more strain on the body. This may create a destructive cycle as the less energy you have, the less you are able to cope with difficult situations.

If nervous exhaustion reaches an extreme, a collapse or breakdown happens which forces you to rest as part of recovery. Stress, anxiety, depression, insomnia, panic attacks, phobias, and overwork may all contribute to nervous exhaustion. Herbs, vitamins C and B-complex, and restful periods can help to fortify the nerves and prevent low vitality.

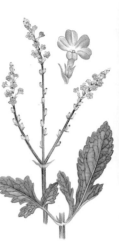

Vervain
(Verbena officinalis)

DANDELION, BURDOCK, AND RED CLOVER

These herbs cleanse your system if your diet has been poor or you have consumed large amounts of caffeine or alcohol. Nettles can also be added to help remineralize your system. Add relaxing herbs such as vervain or lime blossom if symptoms of stress are present.

OATS, VERVAIN, LICORICE, AND SKULLCAP

These herbs help to strengthen the nervous system and support the adrenal glands (often these are overtaxed by stress, overwork, and caffeine). Drink these herbs at least three times daily while avoiding caffeine, alcohol, and tobacco. These are safe to use over a long period.

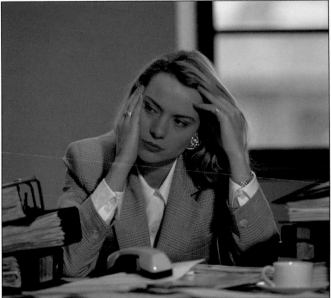

Nervous exhaustion may occur with long-term emotional conflicts, overwork, the over-consumption of tea, coffee, and alcohol, and smoking.

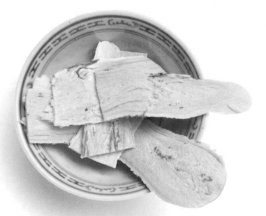

Astragalus
(Radix astragali membranaceus)

Red clover
(Trifolium pratense)

GINSENG AND ASTRAGALUS

These herbs will help to boost physical energy if there is fatigue as well as nervous exhaustion.

THE BACH FLOWER REMEDIES

This is a system of 38 remedies made from the flowers of plants, shrubs, and trees, almost all of which grow wild in North America. The remedies are prepared by soaking the flowers in spring water and letting them sit in the sun. Other than brandy, which is used to preserve the flowers, no other ingredients are used. Though they are not strictly herbs, they are included in this book because they are also derived directly from plants, and because they are easy and safe to self-prescribe.

DR. EDWARD BACH

The flower remedies were evolved by Dr. Edward Bach, a physician and homeopath, who in 1930 gave up his successful London practice to develop his healing work using plants.

It is said that he developed great sensitivity, and that by holding a plant in his hand he had such a strong perception of its energy that he sensed its properties in himself.

Dr. Edward Bach (1886 - 1936)

HOW TO PRESCRIBE

The flower remedies are prescribed according to states of mind, moods, and personality traits; it does not follow that they are not effective for physical problems, but rather they can be seen as affecting the body through the mind. Up to six or seven remedies can be mixed together, though they may also be taken singly. The 38 remedies cover a remarkable range of emotional states: they can be used to help someone recover from shock or trauma (see Rescue Remedy, right), give us confidence before interviews or examinations, and even enable us to get over jetlag more quickly! They are completely safe for old and young, pregnant women, and animals. Plants also benefit from them – never throw away unwanted mixtures of remedies; give them to your plants, which should thrive and flourish as a result!

PREPARATION AND DOSAGE

10ml dropper bottles of the remedies – known as "stock" bottles – are available from many health-food stores and herbal suppliers. For immediate or emergency use, the remedies should be taken in a small quantity of water, although they may be taken directly from the stock bottle if necessary; this is not recommended for long-term use, however, because of the amount of brandy that the patient will ingest! If you need to take the remedy or remedies over a period of time, obtain a 1-ounce dropper bottle from a pharmacy and fill it nearly to the top with spring water. Add two drops of each of your chosen remedies, and, if you wish, a spoonful of brandy to preserve the mixture. (It will last about three weeks without the brandy, perhaps longer if you keep it in the refrigerator.)

Take four drops at least four times a day, either in a drink or directly on the tongue, taking care not to touch the dropper with your tongue or the mixture may become cloudy as a result. When dealing with intense feelings, you can take the remedies more often: every 15 or 20 minutes is fine.

COMBINATIONS

The most widely known combination of Bach remedies is the Rescue Remedy; it is available already made up in stock bottles from most herbal or health-food suppliers. It contains five different flower essences: star of Bethlehem, for shock; rock rose, to help deal with panic; impatiens, for tension and impatience; cherry plum, for the fear of losing control; and clematis, to help focus the mind and prevent fainting. Its possible uses are many: after physical or emotional shock, during a panic attack or near-accident, or after receiving bad news. It will calm children waking with night terrors or bad dreams. Rescue Remedy is also available as an ointment, known as Rescue Cream, which is for external use on lesions, rashes, burns, etc.

Other combinations are based on individual circumstances, and you will need to mix them up yourself: for jet-lag, for example, try the Rescue Remedy with the addition of walnut (for change) and scleranthus (which is grounding). Keep taking the mixture frequently until you are accustomed to the new time zone. A number of remedies are helpful before tests or interviews: larch builds confidence, white chestnut frees the mind of worrying thought, scleranthus helps with decision-making, aspen keeps fears at bay, and impatiens may prevent you from rushing.

As you become familiar with the flower remedies, you will make up your own combinations – the complete safety of this system, even for babies and young animals, means that you can explore its possibilities on yourself, friends, and family without risk, as long as you dilute the remedies well for younger patients.

Some people are sceptical about the power of the Bach flower remedies, but herbalists have had some remarkable results through using them, often with people who had not responded to other methods or whose symptoms had become chronic. They work on the level of very subtle energies, which makes their use difficult to subject to laboratory testing, but may also explain their effectiveness.

RESCUE REMEDY

The most widely known combination of Bach remedies. It contains five different flower essences:

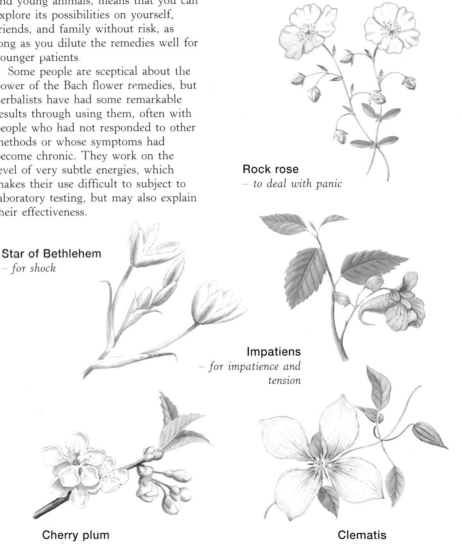

Rock rose
– to deal with panic

Star of Bethlehem
– for shock

Impatiens
– for impatience and tension

Cherry plum
– for fear of losing control

Clematis
– to help focus the mind and prevent fainting

THIRTY-EIGHT REMEDIES

AGRIMONY

For those who use a cheerful exterior to disguise their inner pain.

ASPEN

Allays fears which are vague or unconscious in origin; fears of the intangible, or of death.

BEECH

Encourages tolerance in those who are arrogant or critical of others (may be a temporary state).

CENTAURY

For those who feel unassertive, weak-willed, or imposed upon by others; this remedy helps them determine and realize what they want.

CERATO

Relates to inner certainty; helps people who doubt their own judgment and constantly seek advice.

CHERRY PLUM

Provides reassurance for those who feel they may be on the verge of a breakdown, or "going out of my mind."

CHESTNUT BUD

Helps people to learn by their mistakes; for those who find it hard to become wiser through experience, or who repeat old patterns.

CHICORY

Enables you to let go: for those who are overpossessive of loved ones.

CLEMATIS

Aids concentration in those that are dreamy, unfocused, or vague.

CRABAPPLE

Known as "the cleanser"; helpful for shame, negative feelings about self, after rape or abuse. Often effective for hay fever or rhinitis.

ELM

Relates to responsibility; helpful for those who take on more than they can deal with and become overwhelmed.

GENTIAN

Restores faith in the process of life. Useful for despondency or depression, when the cause is known.

GORSE

Restores hope for those who have given up; despair or chronic illness may be part of the picture.

HEATHER

For those obsessed with their own problems; helps develop compassion.

HOLLY

For rage, jealousy, anger, or any negative emotion; paradoxically, it also helps you contact your true feelings when you feel "cut off."

HONEYSUCKLE

For those nostalgic for the past, honeysuckle will enable letting go and embracing the present.

HORNBEAM

Restores energy when you feel temporarily unmotivated, or procrastinate; often called the "Monday morning" remedy.

IMPATIENS

For impatience and irritability; people who find it hard to work in a team because of these qualities may benefit.

LARCH

Enhances self-confidence and helps you overcome feelings of inferiority or fear of failure.

MIMULUS

Helps deal with fears of known or tangible things, gives courage in the case of phobias.

MUSTARD

Helps reinstate optimism in people who experience sudden depression without a known cause.

OAK

Relates to strength and endurance; for those who overachieve or set themselves impossibly high goals.

OLIVE

Regenerates peace and balance after long periods of overwork or emotional exhaustion.

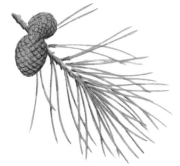

PINE

Helps you to forgive yourself; useful for those with an over-developed sense of guilt.

RED CHESTNUT

Relates to compassion and solicitude; helpful for people who are obsessive about their concern for others, to the point where they project all their own fears onto them.

ROCK ROSE

Reassures where there is panic, terror, or sudden alarm.

ROCK WATER

Not actually a flower, but derived from spring water in natural locations, this remedy frees up people who keep themselves under rigid self-control or self-denial.

SCLERANTHUS

Grounding, helps us make decisions and allays uncertainty or mood swings.

STAR OF BETHLEHEM

Reassures after shock or trauma, sudden loss, or accident.

SWEET CHESTNUT

Helps release the user from a state of hopeless despair.

VERVAIN

Restores balance to the person who expends energy in over-enthusiasm or fanatical beliefs; has a gentle sedative action.

VINE

Relates to qualities of authority and leadership; in the negative vine state, a person may be controlling, ruthless, and power-hungry.

WALNUT

A protective remedy, helping you through periods of transition or gateways; walnut facilitates change

WATER VIOLET

Relates to humility – indications include withdrawn behavior, deliberate isolation – the person is reserved and proud.

WHITE CHESTNUT

Dispels persistent unwanted thoughts; often used for insomnia.

WILD OAT

Helps people find their true direction, purpose, or career, and thus fulfillment.

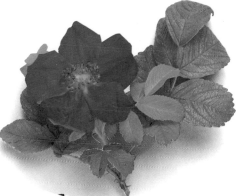

WILD ROSE

Recreates motivation for those who are apathetic or resigned.

WILLOW

Helps give you a sense of personal responsibility: someone in a negative willow frame of mind feels bitter, like a victim, and blames others.

Consulting a Herbal Practitioner

Having developed an interest in herbs, you may wish to enlist the advice and experience of a qualified herbalist; or you may find your health problem is beyond the scope of this book. (Potentially serious ailments, such as asthma, tumors, or heart conditions, have not been included because they obviously require the attention of a professional). You should also bear in mind that some herbs, like some foods, may cause an allergic reaction in sensitive people; if you experience new symptoms while taking herbs, you are strongly recommended to consult a reputable practitioner who will be able to identify the problem. You may be lucky enough to find a herbalist through someone who can recommend a practitioner; it is generally reassuring to know something about their reputation and the way they work. Otherwise, you will need to contact one of the organizations which keep registers of practitioners.

If you are feeling adventurous (or maybe just out of curiosity) of if your condition is more serious, you may prefer to consult someone qualified in prescribing Chinese herbs.

Chinese herbs have a well-deserved reputation for tasting unpleasant (though this is not always the case), but they are more powerful and therefore sometimes more effective than Western herbs.

What to expect

Most herbalists will take a fairly detailed case history, and if you have not consulted a complementary therapist before, this can come as something of a surprise. If you've consulted a therapist about psoriasis, you may certainly wonder why they need to know about your bowels! That's because herbalists mostly work in a holistic way, and need to know as much about the workings of your body and mind as possible, in order to determine what is amiss with your energy.

In Chinese medicine, groups of apparently unrelated symptoms are known as syndromes or "patterns of disharmony," and your practitioner will need to identify how this theoretical framework applies to you; this will generally involve taking your pulse and looking at your tongue, both of which provide a valuable source of information about your energy. Many people in Western cultures are a little shy about showing their tongue to a comparative stranger; rest assured that the herbalist is not trying to identify what you had for breakfast, but is looking at the color, shape, and coating of your tongue to help determine a correct diagnosis.

Having prescribed a suitable mixture of herbs for you, the practitioner will either mix up the prescription in tincture form for immediate use, or (more likely with Chinese herbs) write out a prescription for you to obtain. Sometimes the herbalist will send the list of herbs to a herbal supplier to be mixed up and mailed to you, or occasionally you may be given the herbs in powder, tablet, or tincture form. If you live in a city with a sizable Chinese community and your herbalist can write in Chinese characters, you may have the amazing experience of going to a Chinese herbal shop, where you can sit and wait, surrounded by jars of extraordinary-looking substances, while the clerk weighs out each of your herbs in hand-held scales and wraps them in paper.

The herbs will need decocting daily; follow the instructions for preparation given you by your herbal practitioner. Unlike Western herbs, Chinese herbs are often decocted twice, so that each packet of herbs lasts two days.

If the herbs are not working...

First, have a close look at your lifestyle and diet to see if there are any bad habits blocking the herbs from doing their job. It is simply unrealistic to expect the subtle, natural energy of herbs to have an effect if you live on hamburgers, never exercise, and smoke 40 cigarettes a day! This is an extreme example of course, but it cannot be overemphasized that herbs work best in a body which is also cared for in other ways. It may be helpful, for instance, to consult a nutritionist to help work out a good diet and supplement any vitamin or mineral deficiencies you may have.

Second, it will be harder for the herbs to work if the energy is blocked somewhere in your body, or if important structures are out of alignment. Seeing an acupuncturist or osteopath can make an enormous difference.

Last, it will be difficult to relieve symptoms which are the result of unresolved emotions; if this is the case, you should find a good counselor or therapist so that you can deal with any emotional blocks, enabling your energy to respond more freely to the herbs.

USEFUL ADDRESSES

HERB SUPPLIERS

The addresses listed are just some of the many herb suppliers in U.S. Check the Yellow Pages for other local suppliers.

Great China Herb Company
857 Washington Street
San Francisco
CA 94108
Tel: 415-982-2195

Haussman's Pharmacy
6th Girard Avenue
Philadelphia
Pennsylvania 19123
Tel: 215-627-2143

Herbal Medicine Chest
25 Huntington Avenue
Boston
Mass
Tel: 617-247-1446

May Way Trading Co.
1338 Cypress Street
Oakland
CA 94607
Tel: 510-208-3113

Meadowbrook Herb Garden
Route 138
Wyoming
Rhode Island 02898
Tel: 401-539-4603

New Life
415 Blue Hill Avenue
Roxbury
Mass
Tel: 617-442-4237

Reevis Mountain School
HC02 Box 1534
Roosevelt
AZ 85545
Tel: 520-467-2675

7 Arrows Herb Farm
346 Oakhill Avenue
Attleboro
Mass 02073
Tel: 508-399-7860

Xie Wenfei
Kenmore Square
520 Commonwealth Avenue
Suite 201
Boston
MA 02215
Tel: 617-536-0292

Zhu Chun-Han
1498 Center New
Boston
Mass
Tel: 617-969-0899

HERBAL ORGANISATIONS

American Botanical Council
P.O. Box 201660
Austin
TX 78720-1660
Tel: 512-331-8868

American Herbalists Guild
Box 1683
Soquel
CA 95073

American Herbal Products Association
P.O. Box 2410
Austin
Texas
Tel: 512-320-8555

American Herbalists Association
P.O. Box 1673
Nevada City
CA 95959

READING LIST

Although this book lists about one hundred herbs, it is intended only as an introduction. If you want to develop your knowledge of herbs and Bach flower remedies, the following books are recommended:

Barnard, J. & M., *The Healing Herbs of Edward Bach* (Bach Educational Programme, Hereford, 1988).

Bach, Dr. E., *The Twelve Healers and Other Remedies* (C. W. Daniel, Essex). Describes all 38 flower remedies.

Bensky, D. and Barlott, R., *Chinese Herbal Medicine – Formulas and Strategies* (Eastland Press, Washington, 1990).

Bensky, D. and Gamble, A., *Chinese Herbal Medicine* – Materia Medica (**Eastland Press,** Washington, 1986).

Campion, K., *A Woman's Herbal* (Century, London, 1987).

Curtis, S., Fraser, R., and Kohler, I., *Neal's Yard Natural Remedies* (Arkana, London, 1988).

Fratkin, J., *Chinese Herbal Patent Formulas* (Institute for Traditional Medicine, Portland, Oregon). Rather detailed for the beginner, but very thorough.

Grieve, Mrs. M., *A Modern Herbal* (Penguin Books, London, 1989).

Hoffman, D., *The Holistic Herbal* (Element, Dorset, 1983). Essential reading for every herbal user.

Lust, J., *The Herb Book* (Bantam, New York, 1986).
This American herbal lists a vast range of herbs; also a useful list of suppliers in the U.S.

McIntyre, A., *The Herbal for Mother and Child* (Element, Dorset, 1992).

McIntyre, A., *Herbs for Common Ailments* (Gaia Books, London 1992). Beautifully illustrated and highly recommended.

Scheffer, M., *Bach Flower Therapy – Theory and Practice* (Thorsons, Northants, 1986). A very clear and positive guide to the flower remedies.

INDEX

Note: Page numbers in *italics* refer to illustrations

PICTURE CREDITS
Key: a=above b=below l=left r=right

Hulton-Deutsch Collection 4, John MacRae-Brown/Ace 5, E. T. Archive 6 a & b, Harry Smith Horticultural Collection 14r, 15r & 16r John Searle/Ace 17r, Image Bank 20r, Max Schnider/Image Bank 21 br, Bard Martin/Image Bank 48 bl, Zephyr Pictures/Ace 49r, Pictor 51ar, David Vance/Image Bank 53ar, Eric Simmons/Image Bank 54, Pictor 55 a, courtesy of the Dr. E Bach Centre 56b.

All other photographs are the copyright of Quarto Publishing plc.

Quarto would like to thank Marle Place Garden & Nursery, Brenchley, Nr Tonbridge, Kent for supplying some of the herbs used on photography

Authors' Acknowledgments
Tamara Kircher would like to thank her children, Ryan and Molly Jo for their interest, understanding and self-sufficiency and Clive for his patience and his computer.

Penny Lowery would like to thank Claire Grey for the loan of books and Eileen Bonner for her patience and her computer!